Natural Foods
from the Tapestry of Life

ACTIVITY BOOK

Natural Foods from the Tapestry of Life is intended solely for informational and educational purposes, and not as medical advise. Please consult a medical or health professional if you have questions about your health.

Copyright © 2025 Nutrition in a Nutshell, LLC. All Rights Reserved. No part of this book may be reproduced, or stored in a retrieval system, or transmitted in any form or by any means, electronic, mechanical, photocopying, recording, or otherwise, without express written permission of the publisher.

First Printing 2025. Printed in the United States of America
ISBN: 979-8-9985183-1-7
Library of Congress Control Number: TBD

Published by Nutrition in a Nutshell, LLC, Amy J. Wing, Founder and Owner
Book Design: Eagle Lady Design Studio, Sandra L. Jones
Cover Illustration: Rima Al Turk, ©Dreamstime.com
Published in Prescott, Arizona, United States of America

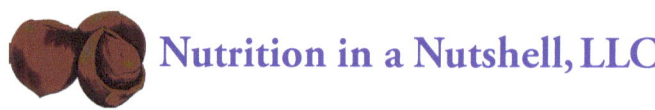

Nutrition in a Nutshell, LLC

NutritioninaNutshell.com
Visit our website to find:

🌱 *Natural Foods from the Tapestry of Life* (ISBN: 979-8-9985183-0-0), referred to as the '*Tapestry* Resource Book' in this **ACTIVITY BOOK**

Nutrition Charts and Natural Foods Sticker Package

These educational materials are designed for educators and anyone studying nature and holistic health

🌱 **Organic, regenerative farm store links to traditional, artisan-prepared natural foods**

Copyright © 2025. All Rights Reserved.

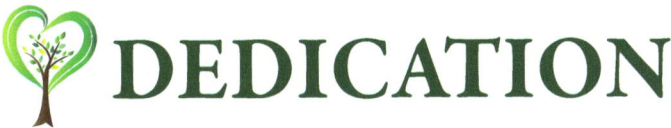DEDICATION

The *Tapestry* books are dedicated to individuals and families who seek the benefits of natural health. Furnishing a compendium of resources, these books describe the high-quality nourishment that can be obtained from traditionally-prepared foods and offer a unique opportunity to study the breadth of natural foods' health-giving properties.

Author Amy J. Wing

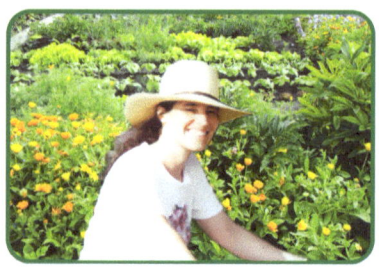

Amy is the founder of Nutrition in a Nutshell, LLC. She has a Master of Science in Health and Nutrition Education degree from Hawthorn University, California, and a Master of Arts in Interdisciplinary Studies degree from George Mason University, Virginia. Amy has 30 years of experience as an ecologist, National Wildlife Refuge System conservation planner, and trainer working for the U. S. Fish and Wildlife Service. Throughout her career, she also worked on family farms in Arizona, Kansas, Maine, Ohio, Scandinavia, Washington, and West Virginia. Amy has studied how the field of natural health has taken shape over the last century and draws on the sound principles of natural healing in writing about natural foods.

Designer and Illustrator Sandra L. Jones

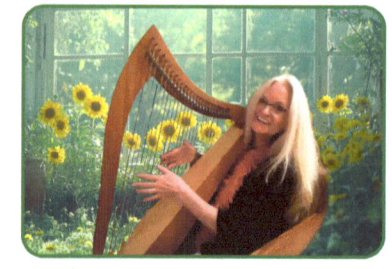

Sandy is an award winning graphic designer. She has successfully designed for authors and businesses for more than four decades, as the designer, illustrator, and owner of Eagle Lady Design Studio. With positivity and confidence, Sandy brings creativity and 'madskillz' to her work for all of her clients. She has an MBA in Marketing, a BA in Graphic Design, and an AA in Fine Art. Additionally, she has completed the UCLA Extension Certificate Program, majoring in Graphic Design, Computer Graphics, and Multimedia. Sandy's vision is for all her clients' designs to unfold as innovative and compelling. She focuses on launching clients' businesses and books from a winning vantage point.

FOREWARD

"As a physician deeply committed to integrative and naturopathic medicine, it's a true honor to write the foreword for this inspiring work. This book is a heartfelt blend of wisdom and science—one that empowers readers to take charge of their health using nature's pharmacy. Amy's passion for holistic wellness shines through every page, offering practical, evidence-informed insights on vitamins, herbs, and healing traditions. It's more than a guide—it's an invitation to reconnect with the body's innate ability to heal."

Your natural partner in health,
Dr. Linda Khoshaba, NMD, FABNE

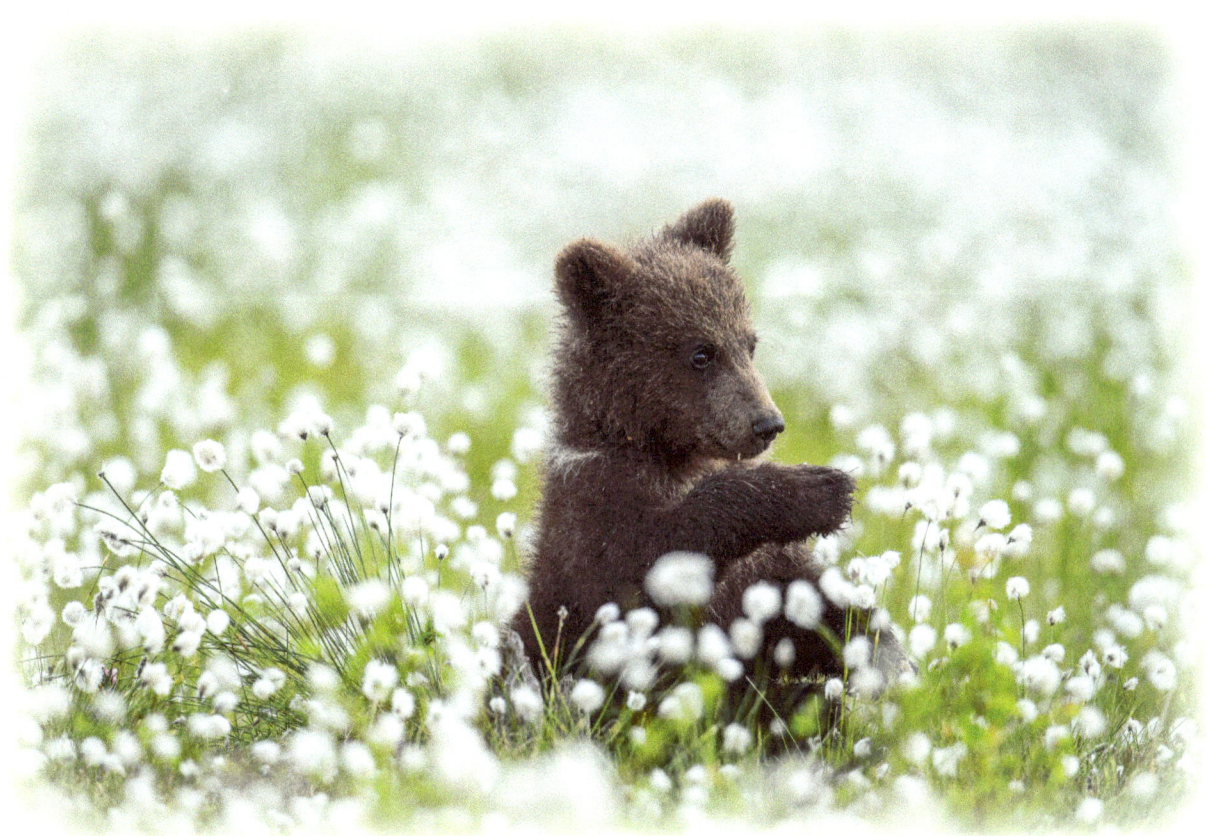

Photographer © Sergey Uryadnikov, Dreamstime.com

Being inquisitive informs us about the world around us
and fosters self-discovery

CONTENTS

How to Use This Book
1

3 Practical Steps
5

21 Educational Activities
9

ACTIVITY BOOK Materials
Landscapes and Seascapes,
Labels, Stickers,
Calendar, Shopping List,
Cookware, Food Processing, and Planters
33

Special Thank You and Acknowledgements 119

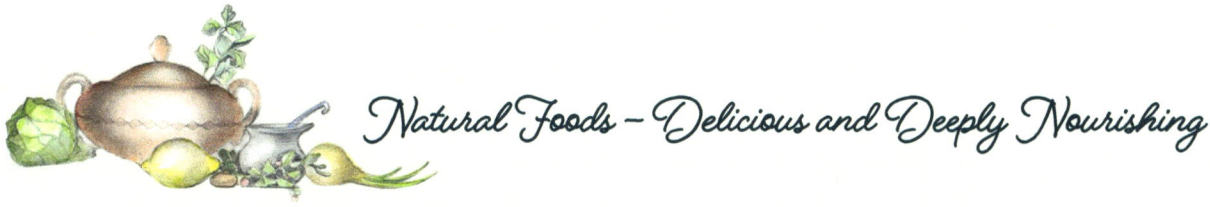

Natural Foods – Delicious and Deeply Nourishing

How to Use This Book

Natural Foods from the Tapestry of Life ACTIVITY BOOK

How to use this ACTIVITY BOOK

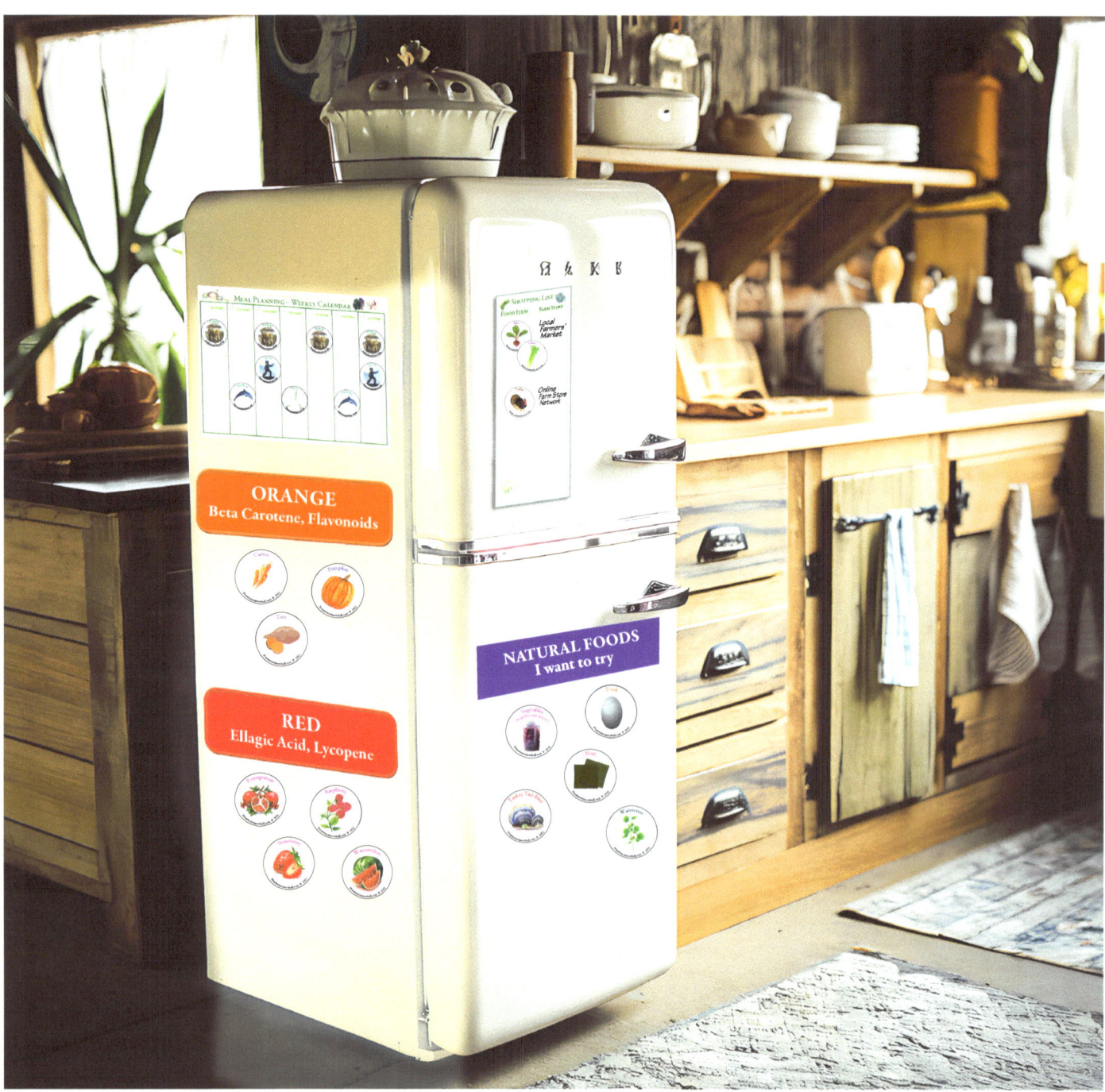

Photographer Hassan Ali, Dreamstime

Example of Activity #11
Colorful & Protective Plant Nutrients

Instructions: Cluster your natural foods (*round stickers*) **by their colorful phytonutrients** (*rectangular stickers*)
(left side of refrigerator)

Example of Activity #1
My Natural Foods New Ones

Instructions: Place the natural foods you want to try (*round stickers*) **under or around the purple label** (*rectangular sticker*)
(right side of refrigerator)

2

Natural Foods from the Tapestry of Life and companion **ACTIVITY BOOK** are designed to engage the interest and imagination of people of all ages in creating nourishing meals with natural foods.

How to use this ACTIVITY BOOK, companion to *Natural Foods from the Tapestry of Life* ('*Tapestry* Resource Book')

Match natural foods (*round stickers*) with their key characteristics (*rectangular sticker labels*) to become familiar with their health-giving benefits.

Peelable, reusable *round stickers* and *rectangular sticker labels* are shown throughout this **ACTIVITY BOOK** and available for purchase at NutritioninaNutshell.com

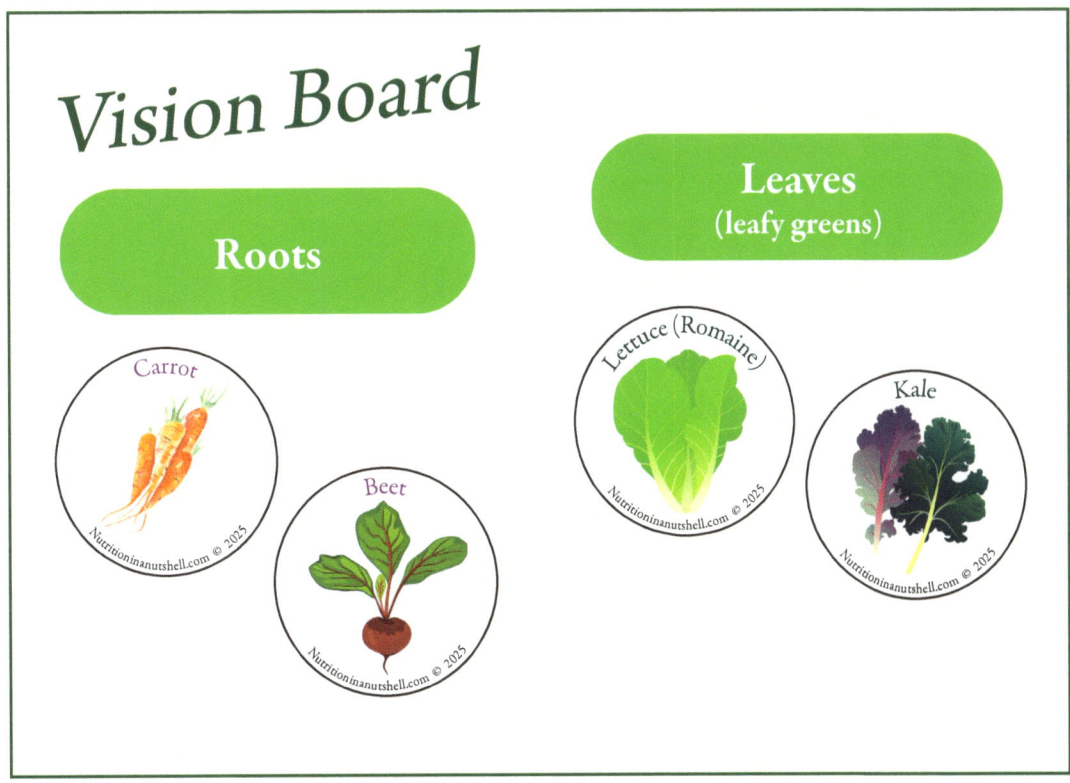

3 Practical Steps

3 Practical Steps

I. What are My Natural Foods?

🌱 **Select your natural foods–Common Food Groups** (*rectangular stickers*, **ACTIVITY BOOK**, shown on page 13) **and/or individual natural foods** (*round stickers*) **and place them on your refrigerator door or vision board**
(ref. *Tapestry* Resource Book, PART I, pages 1 - 23)

> Peelable, reusable *round stickers* and *rectangular sticker labels* are available for purchase at NutritionInaNutshell.com

II. Who are my gardeners, farmers, and wild harvesters?
Including fishing, hunting, foraging

Quality is everything for nutrition & flavor!

Organic, regenerative, humane, pastured, 100% grass-fed, free-range, wild harvested, traditionally prepared

🌱 **Grow and harvest your own natural foods**
(ref. *Tapestry* Resource Book, pages 104 - 111; **ACTIVITY BOOK**, Activity #20, page 29)

🌱 **Find organic, regenerative farm stores near you**
(ref. www.nutritioninanutshell.com/organic-farm-stores-near-you)

🌱 **Find organic, regenerative farm stores that ship throughout the United States and internationally**
(ref. www.nutritioninanutshell.com/farm-store-network)

III. How do I combine my natural foods to make nourishing meals?

🌱 **Plan meals for the week and list meals on your calendar**
(ref. **ACTIVITY BOOK**, page 93;
Tapestry Resource Book, PART IX Planning Nourishing Meals, pages 251 - 287)

🌱 **Complete your shopping list** (ref. **ACTIVITY BOOK**, page 95), **harvest from your garden, and shop at your favorite farm stores**

21 Educational Activities

Educational Activity #1

My Natural Foods
Favorites & New Ones

Instructions: Place your favorite natural foods (*round stickers*) **and the new ones you want to try under or around these two labels** (*rectangular sticker labels*)

My Favorite Natural Foods

NATURAL FOODS **I want to try**

Natural Foods from the Tapestry of Life ACTIVITY BOOK

Educational Activity #2
My Natural Foods
Common Food Groups

Instructions: Choose your natural foods (*round stickers*) **and place them under these Common Food Groups** (*rectangular sticker labels*)

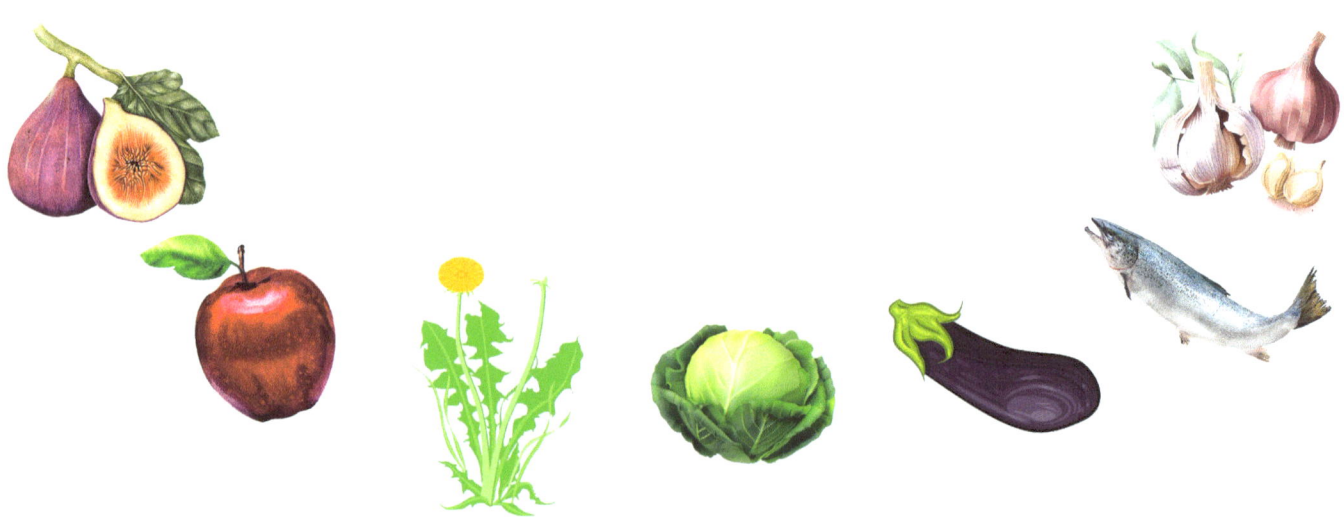

Continued...

Educational Activity #2

Seafoods	Seeds
Meats	Seasonings
Milk Products	Vegetables
Land & Water Fowl Eggs	Leafy Greens
Animal Fats	Plant Oils
Fruits	Mushrooms
Grains	Seaweeds & Chlorella (Algae)
Legumes	Cyanobacteria
Nuts, Bark, Saps	Probiotic Ferments (Bacteria & Micro-Fungi)

Educational Activity #3

My Natural Foods from Five Kingdoms of Life

Instructions: Cluster your Common Food Groups
(*rectangular label stickers,* ACTIVITY BOOK, *shown on page 13*)
under or around these 5 Kingdoms of Life (*rectangular sticker labels*)

(ref. *Tapestry* Resource Book, PART II Foods from Nature, pages 259, 25 - 63)

> *Animalia* **Kingdom**
> (Animal foods)

> *Bacteria* **Kingdom**
> (Probiotic bacteria)

> *Chromista* **Kingdom**
> (Brown algae)

> *Fungi* **Kingdom**
> (Probiotic micro-fungi & mushrooms)

> *Plantae* **Kingdom**
> (Plants, green & red algae)

Educational Activity #4

Examples of Five Plant Families in the *Plantae* Kingdom

Instructions: Cluster your plant foods (*round stickers*) **around these 5 *Plantae* Kingdom families** (*rectangular sticker labels*)

(ref. *Tapestry* Resource Book, PART IV Nutrient Library, pages 124 - 129)

Cruciferous Family
Brassicaceae

Grass Family
Poaceae

Nightshade Family
Solanaceae

Onion Family
Alliaceae

Rose Family
Rosaceae

Educational Activity #5

Botany – Edible Plant Parts

Instructions: Cluster your plant foods (*round stickers*) **by their relevant plant parts** (*rectangular sticker labels*)

(ref. *Tapestry* Resource Book, PART IV Nutrient Library, pages 130 - 138)

- **Roots**
- **Bulbs** (with leaves)
- **Stalks/Stems** (with leaves)
- **Bark**
- **Flowers**
- **Flower Buds**
- **Fruits**
- **Seeds in Pods** (fresh & dried)
- **Seeds** (fresh & dried)
- **Leaves** (leafy greens)

21 EDUCATIONAL ACTIVITIES

Educational Activity #6

Eating by the Seasons

Instructions: Cluster your natural foods (*round stickers*) **by the season when they are harvested in your area** (*rectangular sticker labels*)

(ref. *Tapestry* Resource Book, PART III The Tapestry of Life, pages 104 - 111)

Spring Harvest 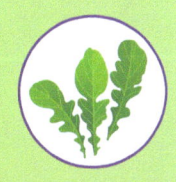   **Summer Harvest**

Autumn Harvest 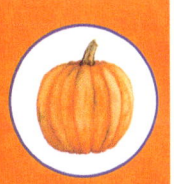   **Winter Harvest and Foods Preserved from Other Seasons**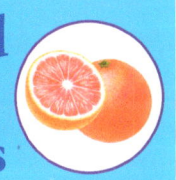

Educational Activity #7
Locally Grown

Instructions: Cluster your natural foods (*round stickers*) **by what is grown in your area** (*rectangular sticker label*)

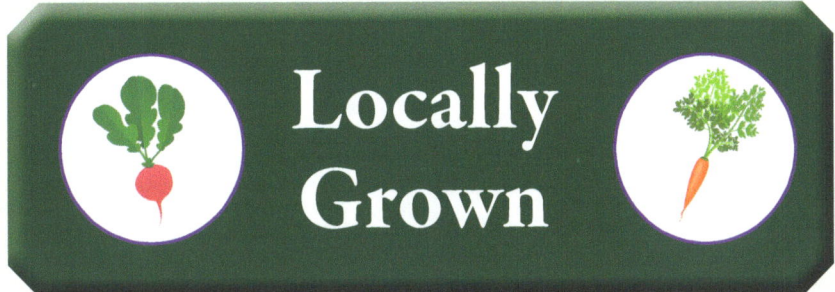

Field Trip Activity
Take field trips during different seasons to see the natural foods growing on local organic, regenerative farms

17

Educational Activity #8
Wild Harvest

Instructions: Cluster the natural foods (*round stickers*) you want to forage and harvest wild in your area (*rectangular sticker label*)

Wild Harvested in your area

Educational Activity #9
Where is the Home of Your Natural Foods?

Instructions: Place your natural foods (*round stickers*) in their ecosystems (habitats) on landscapes and seascapes
(ACTIVITY BOOK, pages 33 -63)

Examples below

(ref. *Tapestry* Resource Book, PART II Foods from Nature, pages 25 - 63)

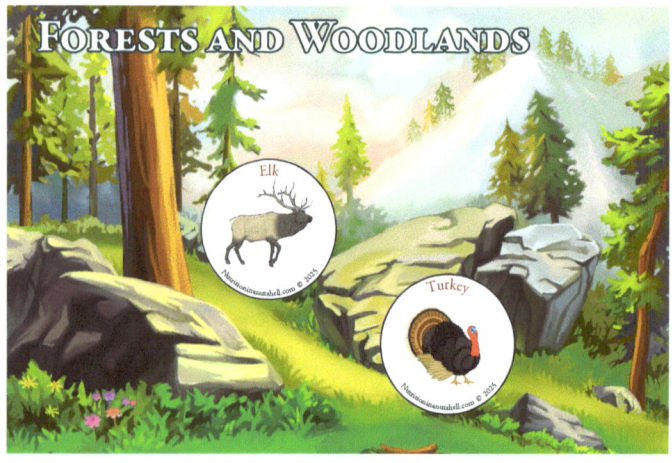
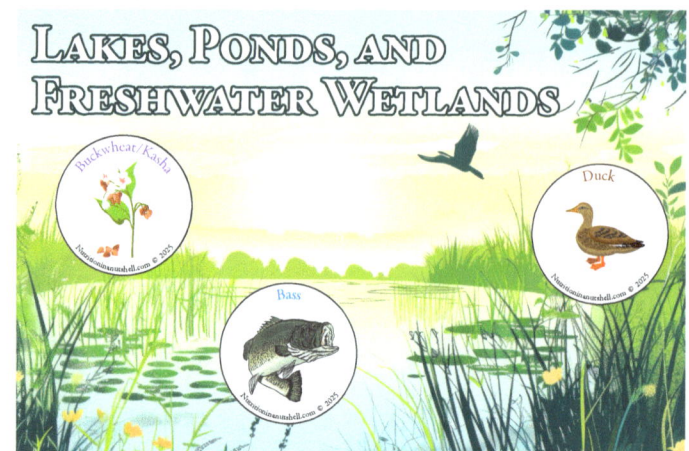

Educational Activity #10
Macro Nutrients

Instructions: Cluster your Common Food Groups (*rectangular sticker labels,* **ACTIVITY BOOK**, shown on page 13) **or individual natural foods** (*round stickers*) **under or around these Macro Nutrients** (*rectangular sticker labels*)

(ref. *Tapestry* Resource Book, PART IV Nutrient Library, pages 154 - 166)

- **ANIMAL** Protein and Lipids (Fats)
- **ANIMAL** Protein and Lipids (Fats) Simple Carbohydrates
- **ANIMAL** Lipids (Fats)
- **PLANT** Simple Carbohydrates
  - Acid Fruits
  - Sub-Acid Fruits
  - Sweet Fruits
  - Melons (sweet)

- **PLANT, FUNGI, & ALGAE** Complex Carbohydrates (Non-starch)
- **PLANT** Complex Carbohydrates (Mild-starch)
- **PLANT** Complex Carbohydrates (Starch)
- **PLANT** Complex Carbohydrates and Protein (Starch and Protein)
- **PLANT** Lipids (Fats and Oils)
- **PLANT** Protein, Lipids (Oils), and Carbohydrates

19

Educational Activity #11
Colorful & Protective Plant Nutrients

Instructions: Cluster your natural food stickers *(round stickers)* **by their colorful phytonutrients** *(rectangular sticker labels)*

(ref. *Tapestry* Resource Book, PART IV Nutrient Library, page 123)

RED
Ellagic Acid, Lycopene

GREEN & WHITE
Indoles, Lutein

ORANGE
Beta Carotene, Flavonoids

GREEN
Chlorophyll, Folate

YELLOW
Kaempferol, Zeaxanthin

BLUE & PURPLE
Anthocyanidins, Pterostilbene

WHITE & GREEN
Allyl Sulfides, Quercetin

RED & PURPLE
Resveratrol, Betacyanin

Educational Activity #12
Foods with Soluble & Insoluble Fiber

Instructions: Cluster your Common Food Groups (*rectangular sticker labels,* ACTIVITY BOOK, *shown on page 13*) **based on whether or not they contain fiber** (*rectangular sticker labels*)

(ref. *Tapestry* Resource Book, PART IV Nutrient Library, page 151 - 153)

With Fiber   **Without Fiber**

Educational Activity #13
Acid & Alkaline-Forming Foods

Instructions: Cluster your Common Food Groups (*rectangular sticker labels,* ACTIVITY BOOK, *shown on page 13*) **or individual natural foods** (*round stickers*) **by Acid-forming, Neutral pH, and Alkaline-forming**

(ref. *Tapestry* Resource Book, PART IX Planning Nourishing Meals, page 253-255)

Acid–Forming   **Neutral pH**

Alkaline–Forming

Educational Activity #14

Anti-Microbial Foods that Support the Immune System

Instructions: Cluster your natural foods (*round stickers*) **that have anti-microbial** (anti-pathogen) **properties under and around the label below** (*rectangular sticker label*)

(ref. *Tapestry* Resource Book, PART VI 11 Systems, page 196)

Anti-Microbial

Educational Activity #15

My Natural Food Goals

Instructions: Identify your natural food goals and objectives

My Natural Food Goals _____

_____

_____

_____

_____

_____

My Natural Food Objectives

Instructions: Complete Activity #16 (page 24) first and do research as needed to set your objectives below

Eat _____ per _____
    _{Number/quantity of a particular Common Food Group}   Time Period
    _{(*rectangular sticker label*) **or** natural food (*round sticker*)}

Eat _____ per _____

Eat _____ per _____

Eat _____ per _____

Eat _____ per _____

Eat _____ per _____

Eat _____ per _____

Eat _____ per _____

Eat _____ per _____

Eat _____ per _____

Eat _____ per _____

Eat _____ per _____

Educational Activity #16
Design Your Own Activity

Instructions: Identify nutrients you want to emphasize for your health and place your natural foods (*round stickers*) that are a good source of these nutrient(s) in the forms on the next page

(ref. *Tapestry* Resource Book, PART IV Nutrient Library, pages 119 - 210)

Example

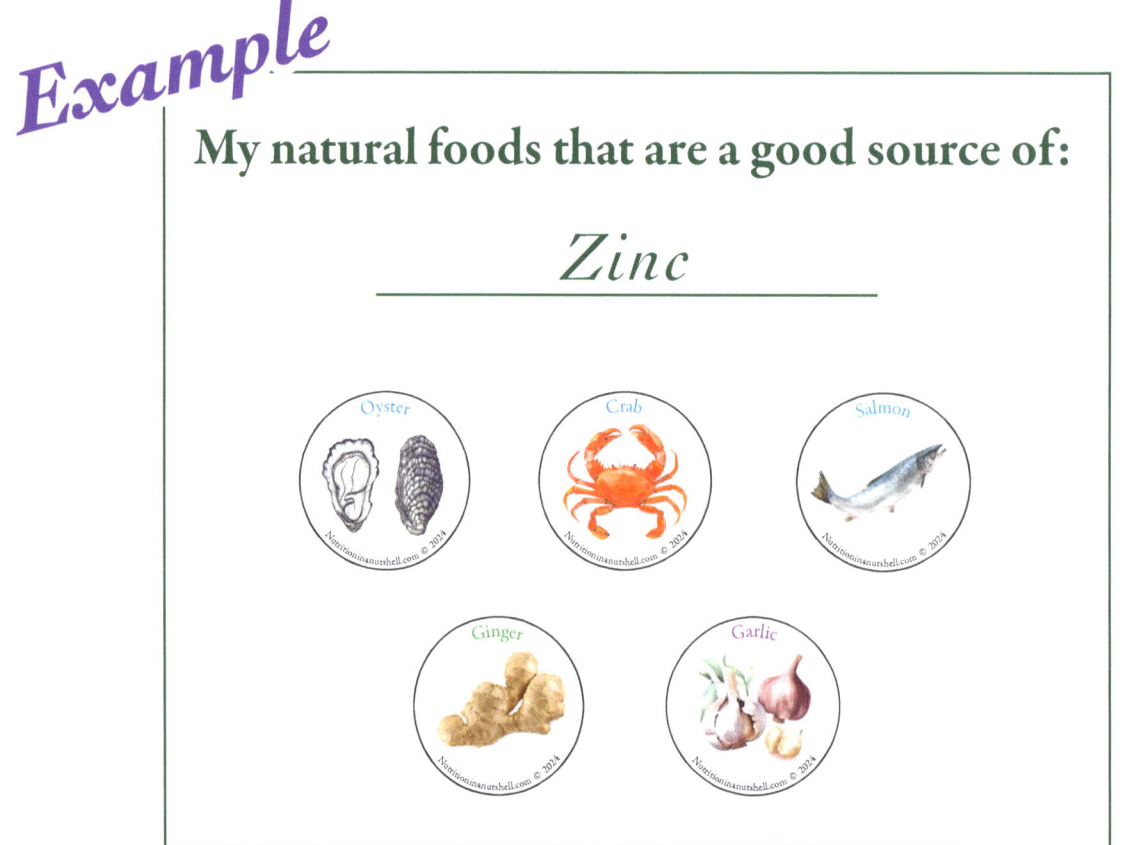

Research idea: identify associated nutrients needed by the body to utilize the nutrient(s) you selected

(for example, bioflavinoids are needed to assimilate vitamin C)

21 EDUCATIONAL ACTIVITIES

My natural foods that are a good source of:

_____

My natural foods that are a good source of:

_____

Natural Foods from the Tapestry of Life ACTIVITY BOOK

Educational Activity #17
Tastes of Natural Foods

Instructions: Notice the distinctive tastes and aromas of different natural foods and cluster them (*round stickers*) **under or around these 6 tastes** (*rectangular sticker labels*)

(ref. *Tapestry* Resource Book, PART IX Planning Nourishing Meals, page 252)

SWEET	**BITTER**
SALTY	**PUNGENT**
SOUR	**ASTRINGENT**

21 EDUCATIONAL ACTIVITIES

Educational Activity #18
Traditionally-Prepared
Homemade & Artisan-Made

Instructions: Cluster your natural foods (*round stickers*) **by Traditionally-Prepared Methods** (*rectangular sticker labels*)

(ref. *Tapestry* Resource Book, PART IX Planning Nourishing Meals, pages 259 - 285)

Slow Cook Stocks and Bone Broths (page 264 - 265)	Soak and Sprout Seeds, Nuts, Grains, Legumes (pages 270 - 272)
Marinate Natural Foods (page 260, 280)	Ferment Natural Foods (pages 282 - 283)

Cook Mushrooms (page 277 - 278)

Preparing Natural Foods in the Kitchen

Place your natural foods (*round stickers*) in the cookware and kitchen appliance illustrations (**ACTIVITY BOOK**, pages 97 - 111)

Examples Below

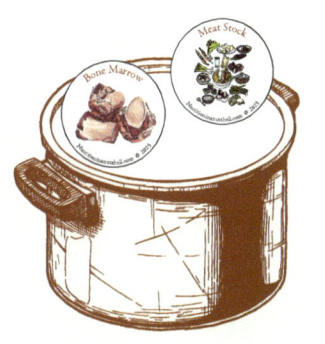
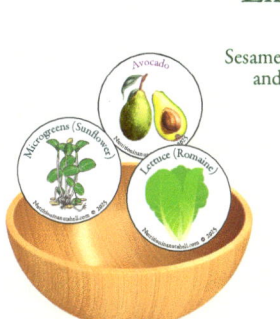
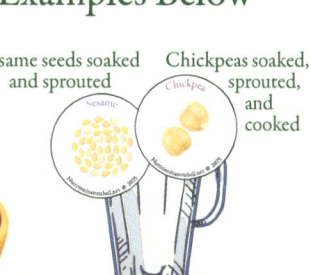
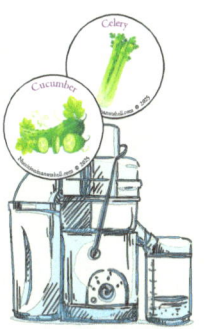
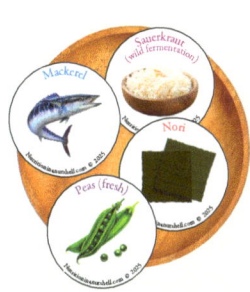

Natural Foods from the Tapestry of Life ACTIVITY BOOK

Educational Activity #19

Plan Ahead for Traditionally Preparing Your Natural Foods

Instructions: Place your natural foods to be traditionally-prepared (*round stickers*) **on your calendar** (ACTIVITY BOOK, shown on pages 88, 93)

(ref. *Tapestry* Resource Book, PART IX Planning Nourishing Meals, pages 259 - 285)

Preparing Natural Foods Traditionally

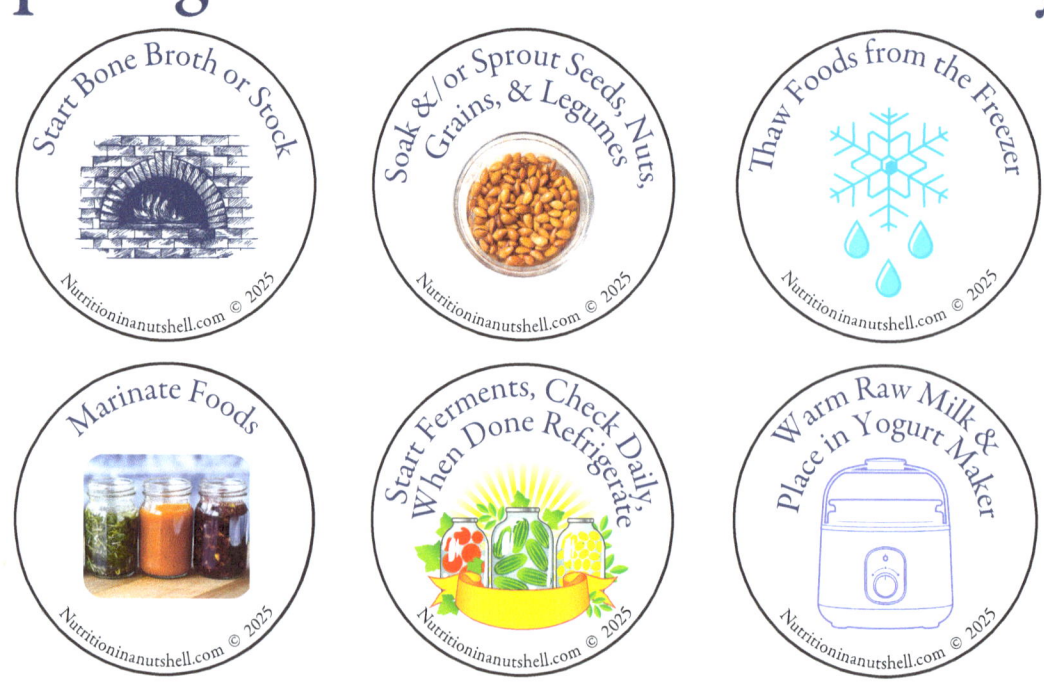

Educational Activity #20
Planning Your Natural Foods Garden

What natural foods would you like to grow and harvest in your raised bed, clay pot, or window box?

Instructions: Cluster your natural foods (*round stickers*) **within the clay pot, window box, and raised bed** (**ACTIVITY BOOK**, pages 113, 115, 117)

(ref. *Tapestry* Resource Book, PART III The Tapestry of Life, pages 104 - 109)

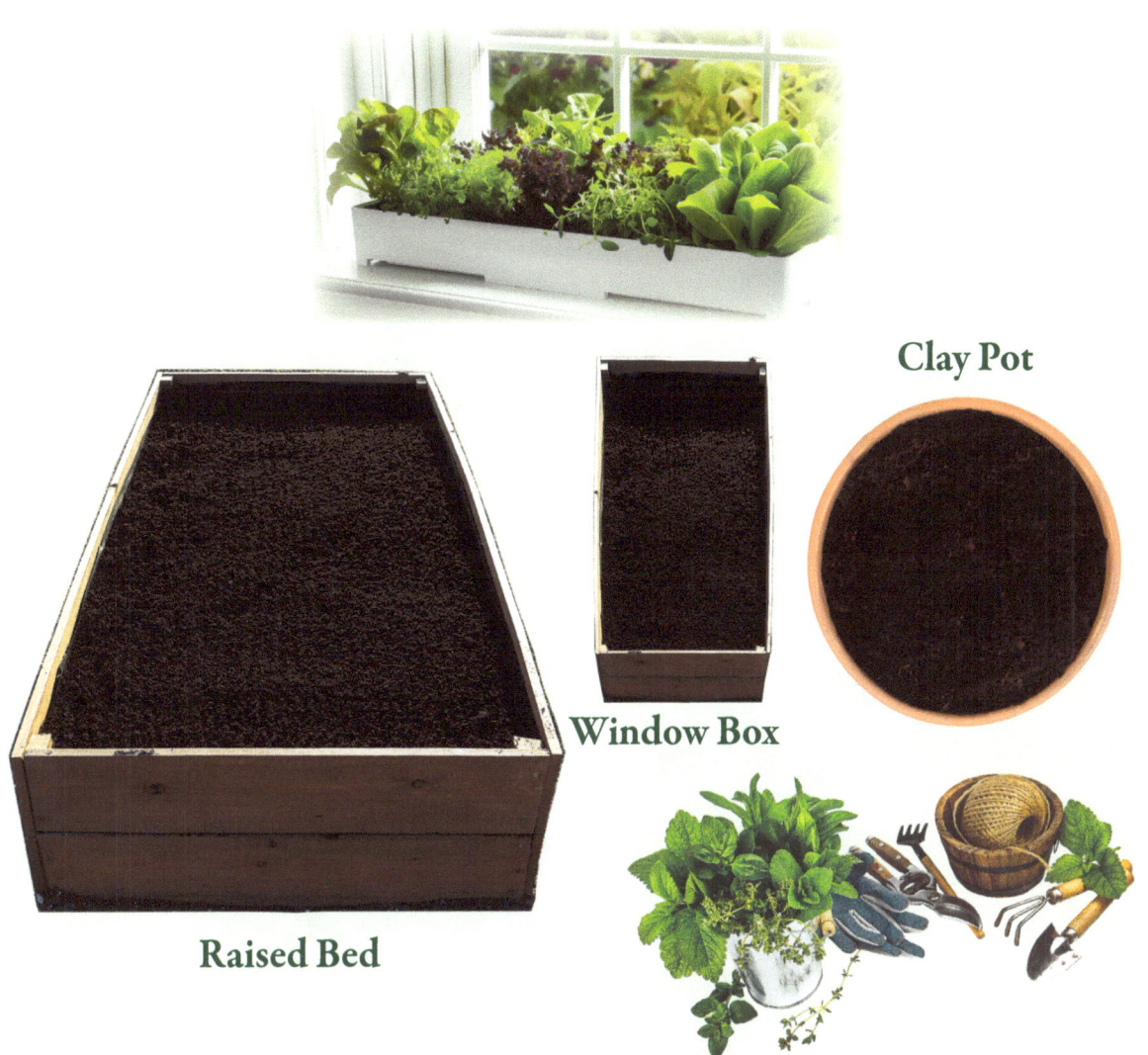

Clay Pot

Window Box

Raised Bed

Educational Activity #21

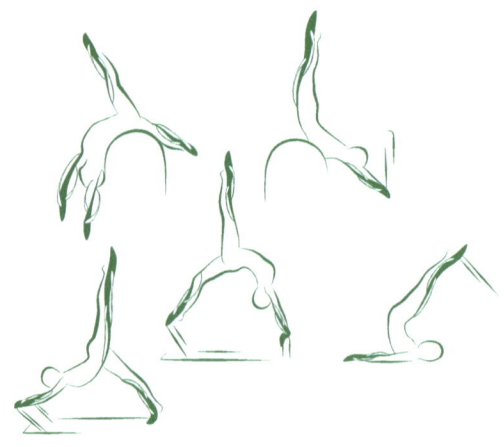

Physical Activities

What physical activities are fulfilling and bring you joy?

Instructions: Place your natural living stickers (*round stickers*) (**ACTIVITY BOOK**, shown on page 89) **on your calendar** (page 93)

(ref. *Tapestry* Resource Book, PART VIII Natural Living, pages 230 - 238)

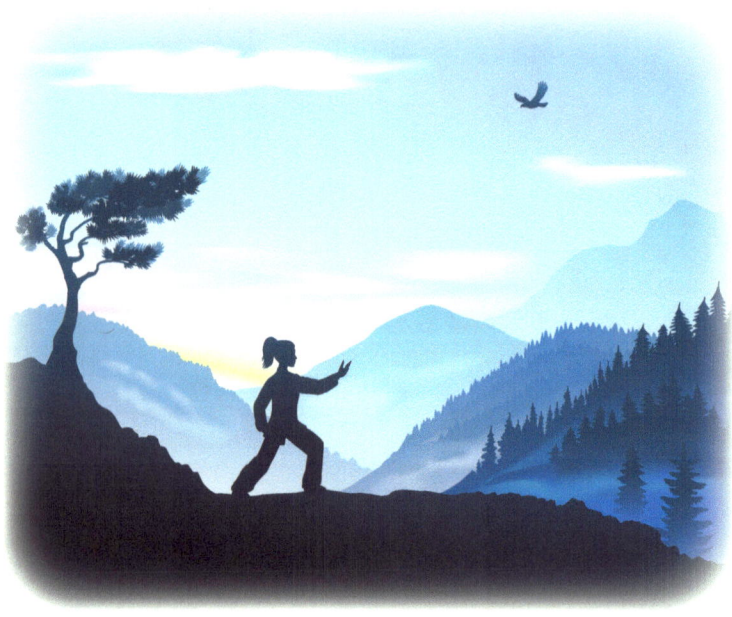

With great appreciation to the Artists who contributed to these landscape and seascape photos and illustrations at ©Dreamstime.com

Photographer:
Desert Scene Photo by Alexey Stiop

Illustrators:
Forests and Woodlands by Nextmars
Deciduous Forests by Elena Mikhaylova
Tropical Forests by Sabrina Sultana
Boreal Snow Forests and Rivers by Sabrina Sultana
Grasslands and Meadows by Czibo
Lakes, Ponds, and Freshwater Wetlands by Svetlana Leuto
Bayous by Saiful Islam
Mangroves by Satori13
Estuaries by Stockeeco
Sand Dunes and Coastal Waters by Oiiobas
Coast and Ocean Floor by Olga Kurbatova
Deep Ocean by S-dmit
Deserts and Mountains by Woranuch Athiwatakara
Gardens and Farms by Athiphat Tanglukdee
Regenerative, Organic Markets by Alexandrepatchine

A Closer Look at Ecosystems on Landscapes & Seascapes

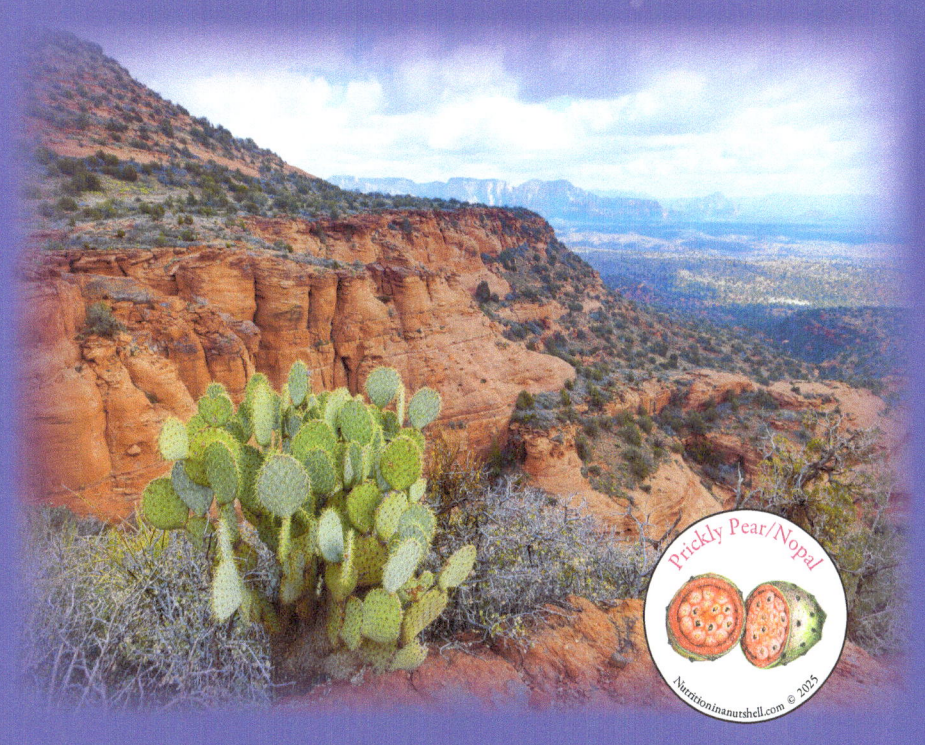

Forests and Woodlands
Meadows
Lakes, Streams, and Wetlands
Estuaries, Coasts, and Oceans
Deserts
Farms and Markets

Place your natural foods (*round stickers*) where they are found in their natural, garden, or farm habitats

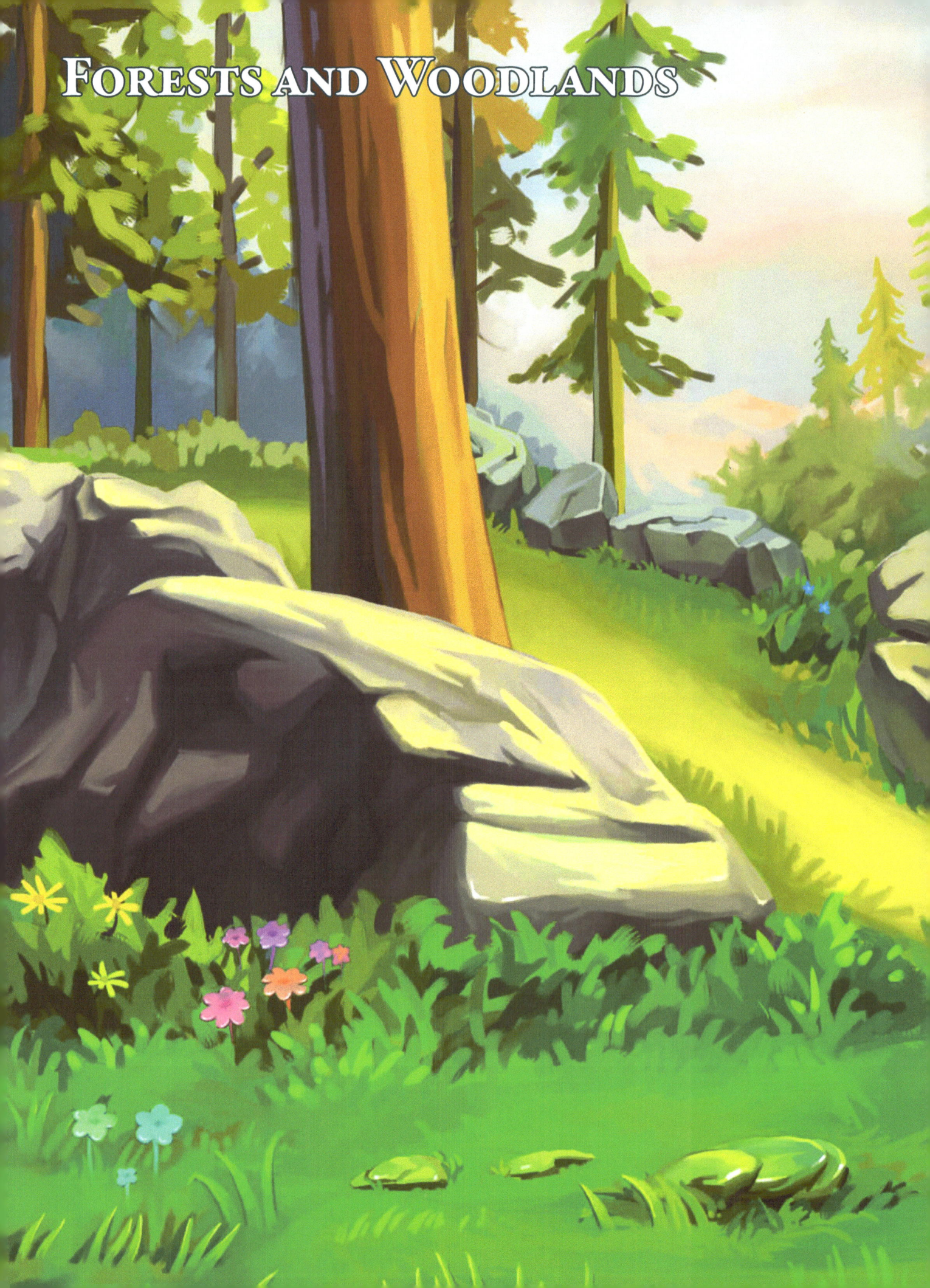

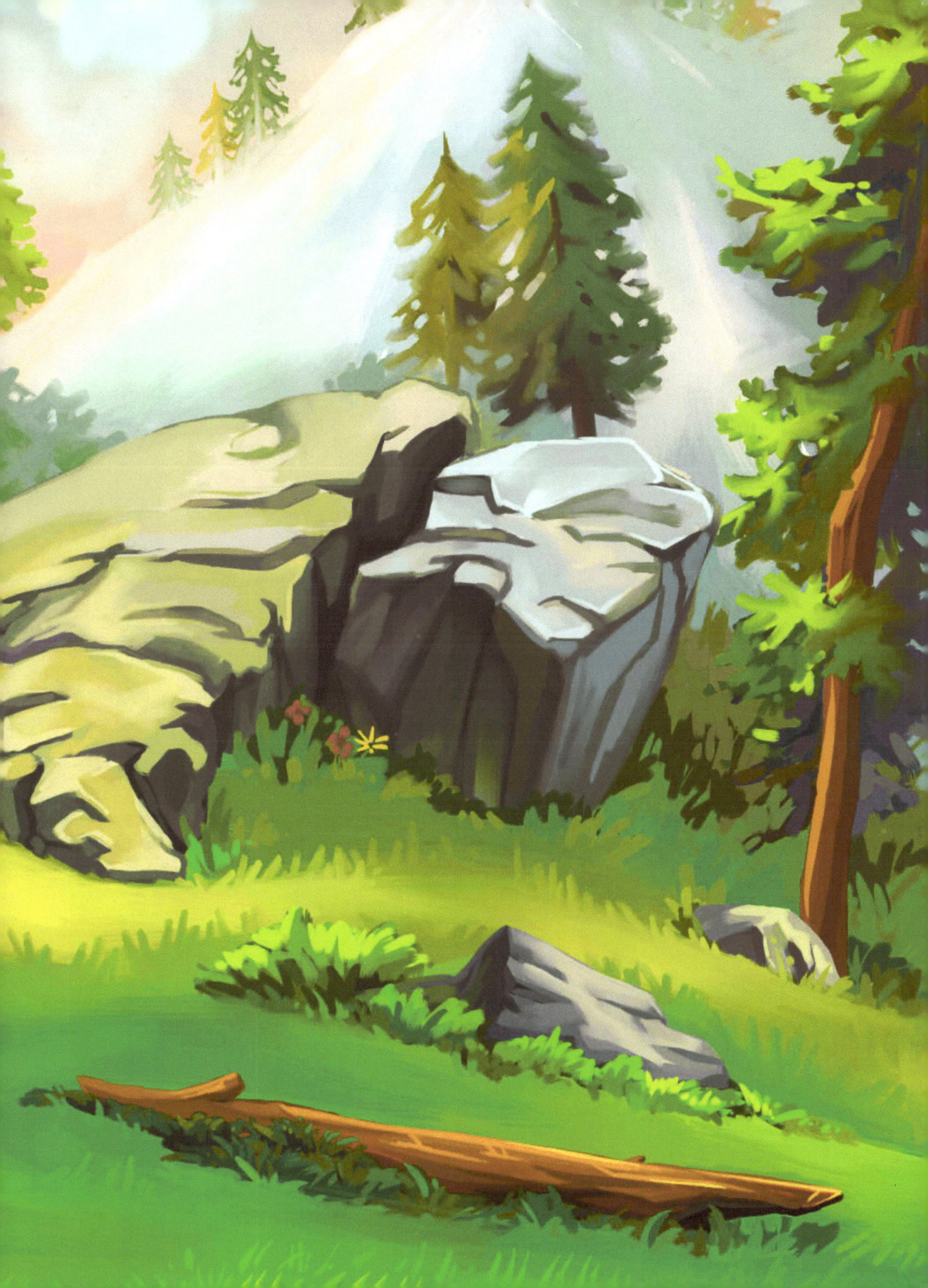

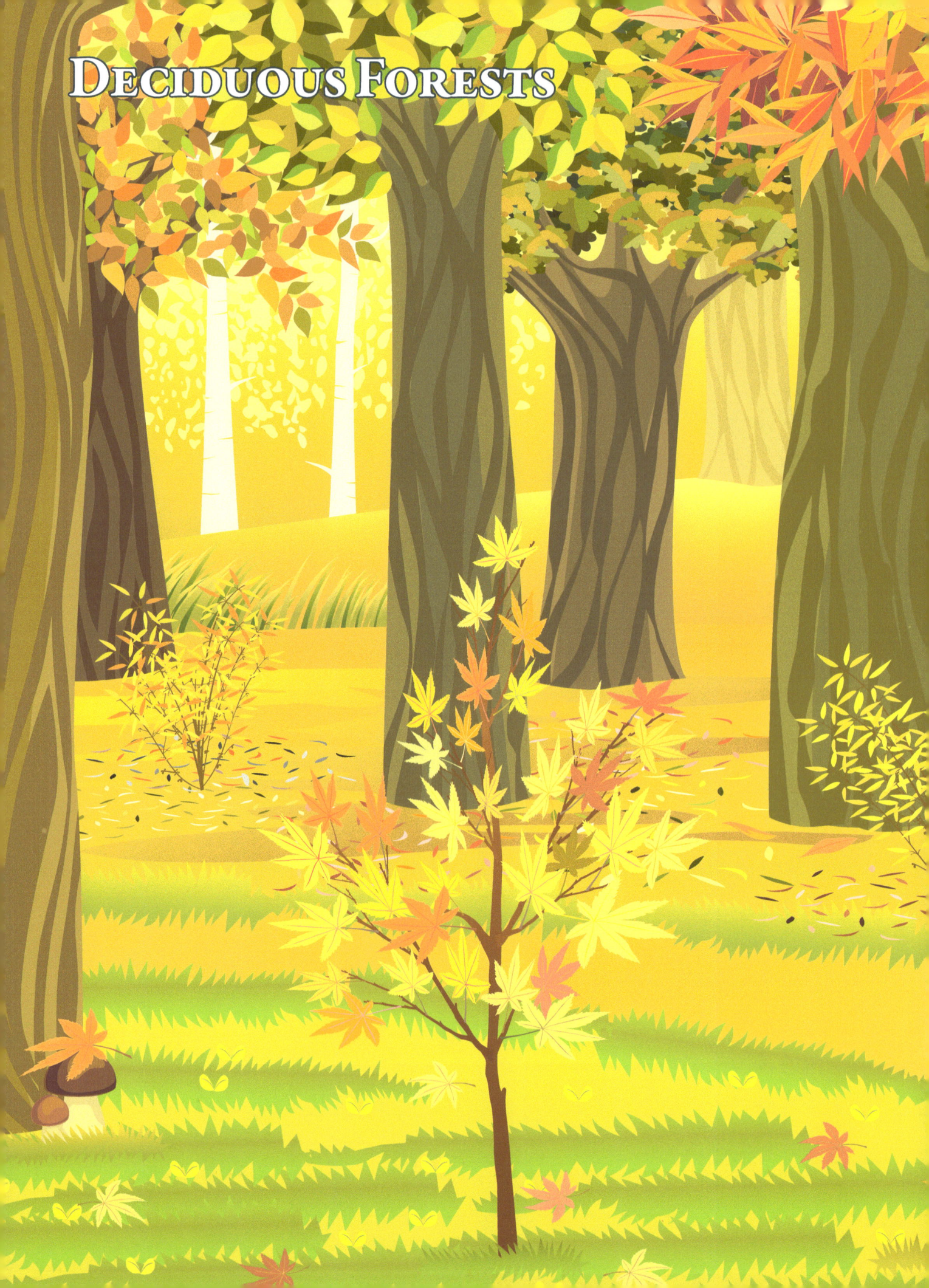

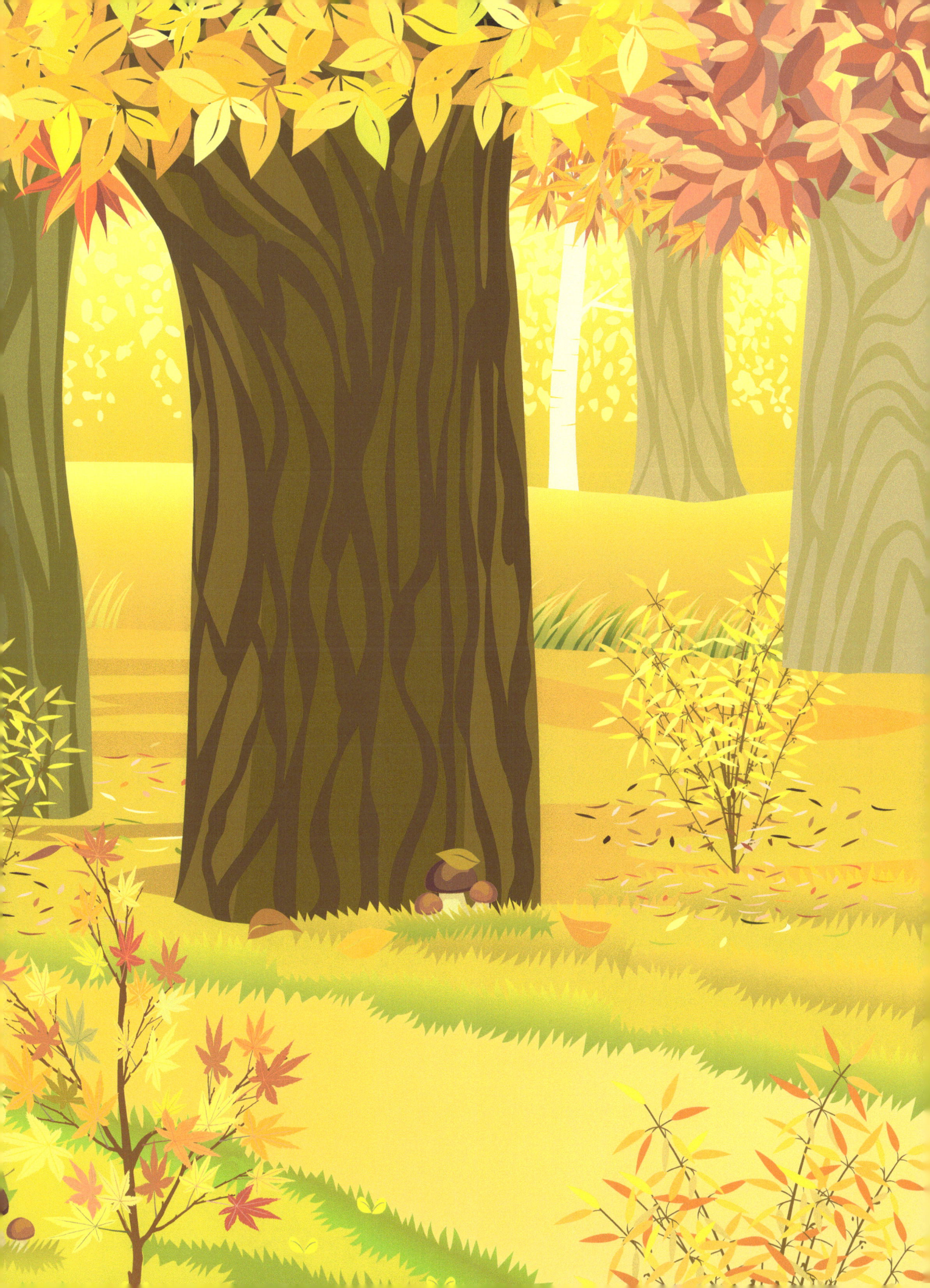

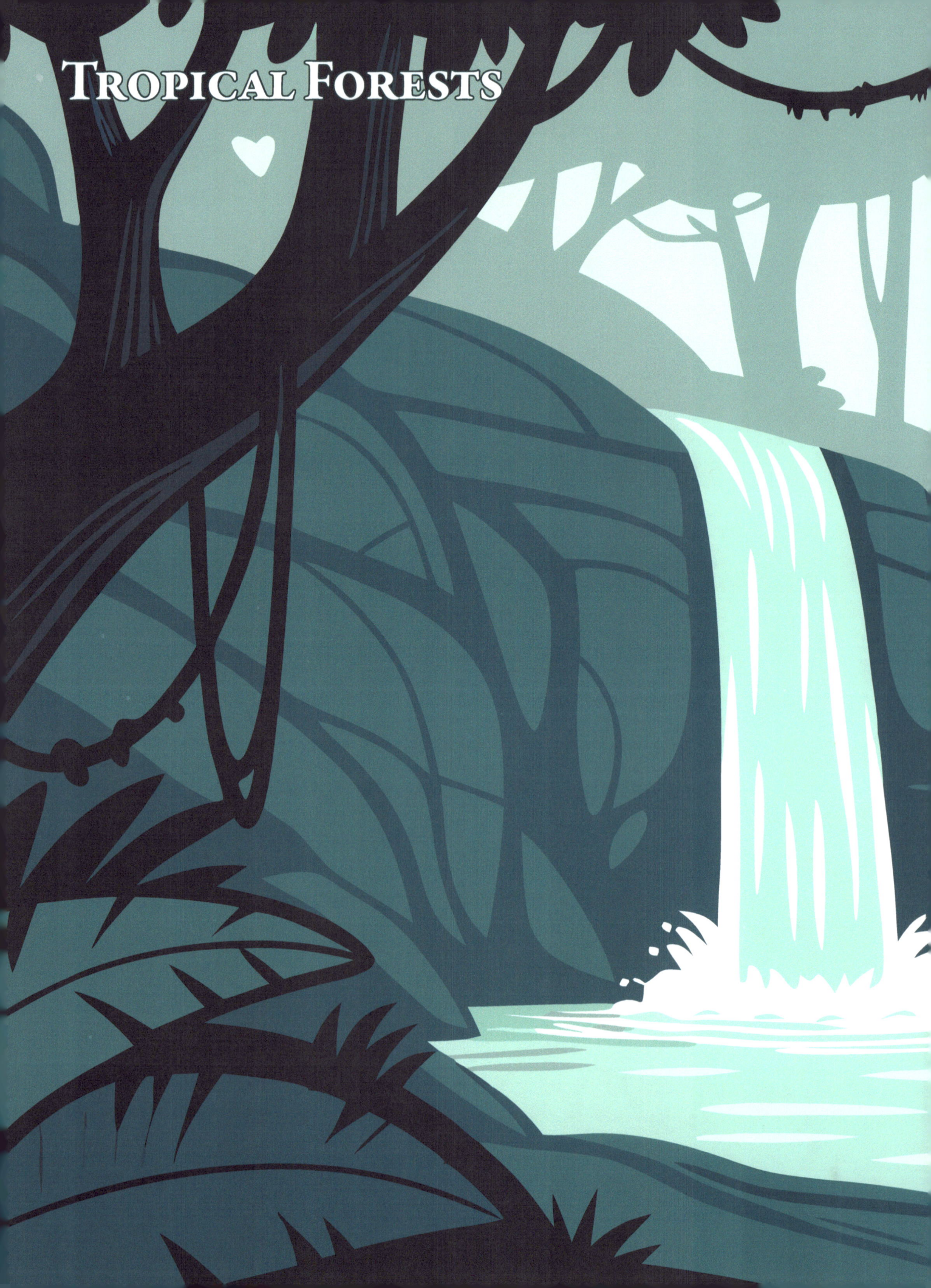

Tropical Forests

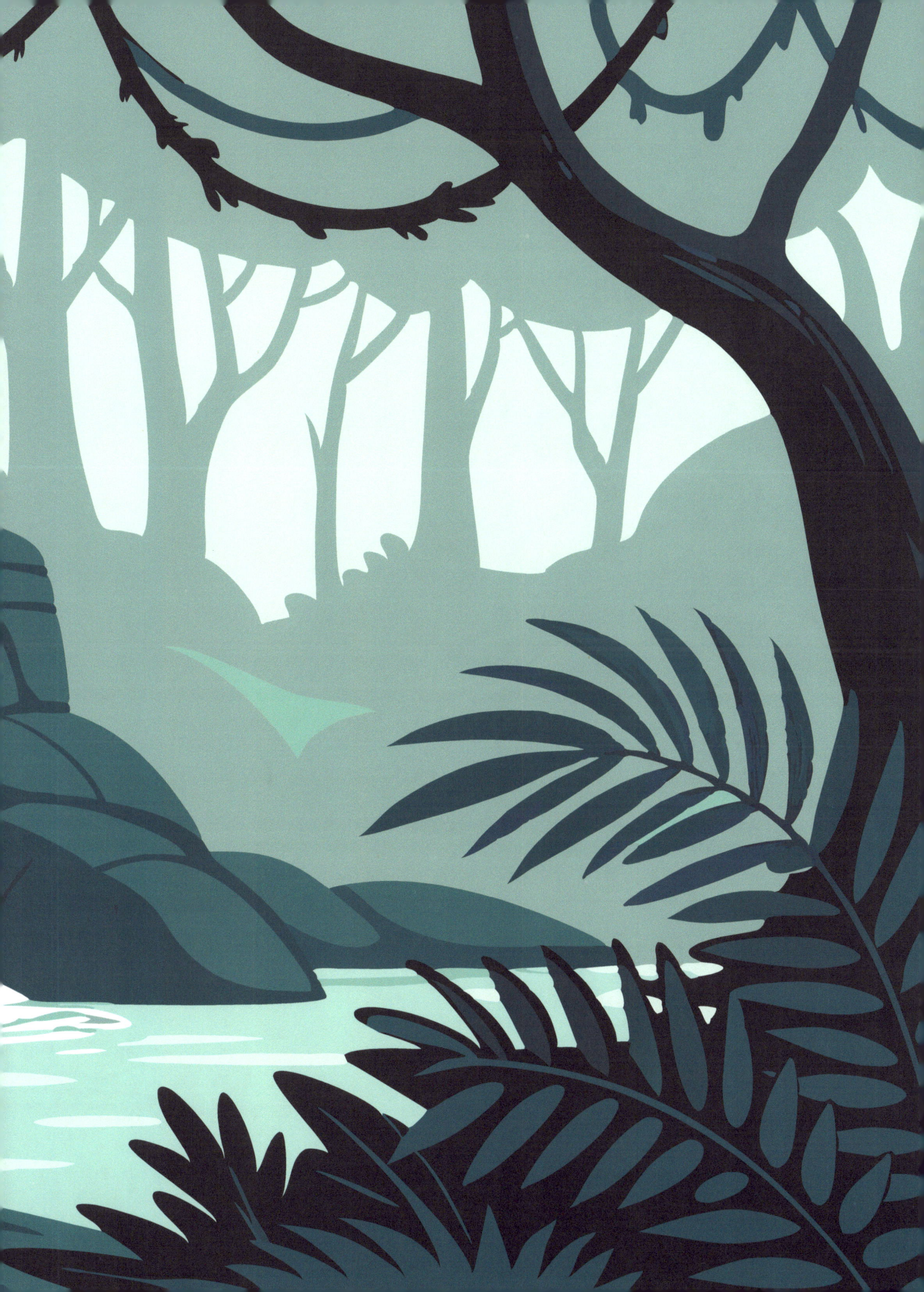

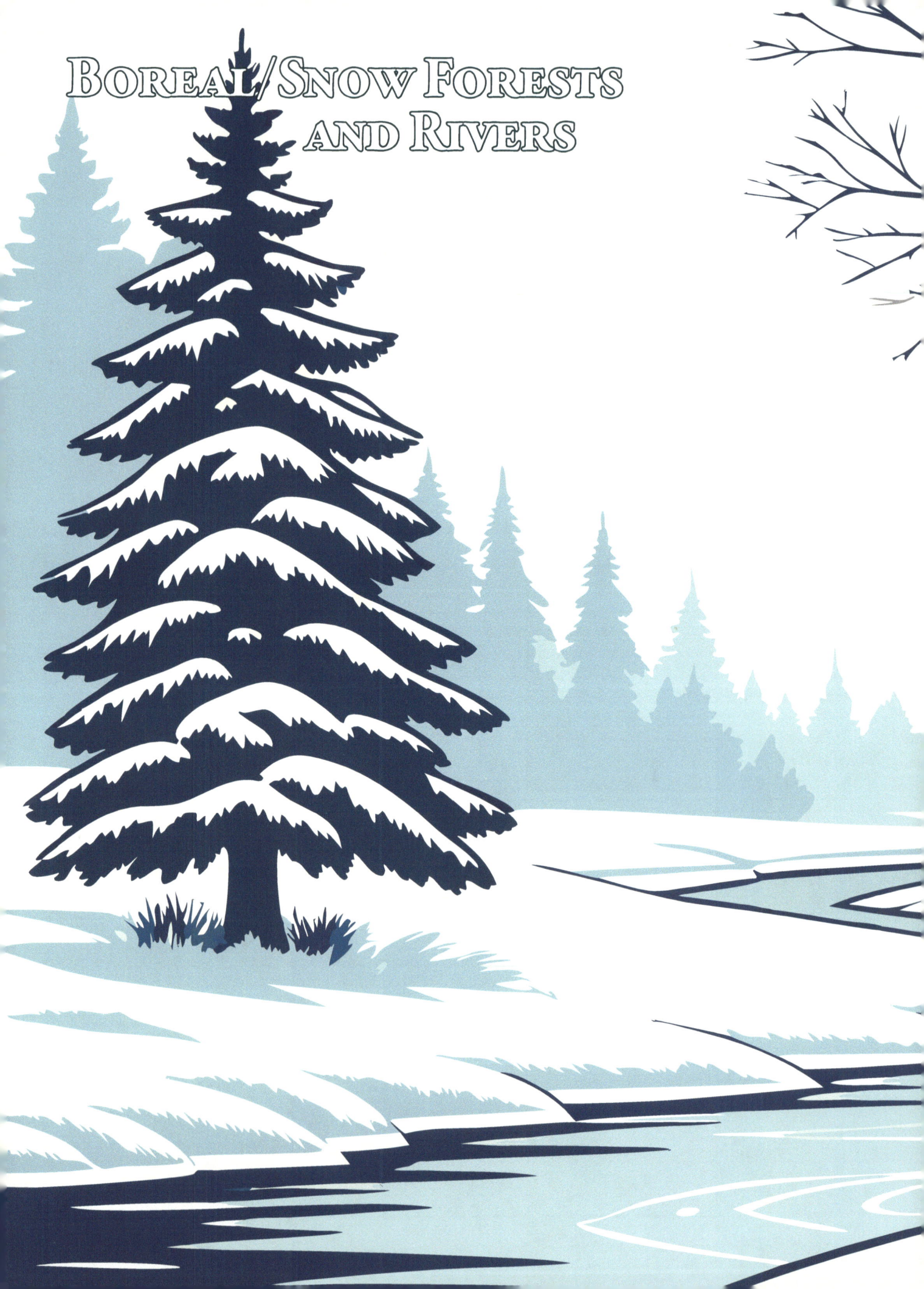

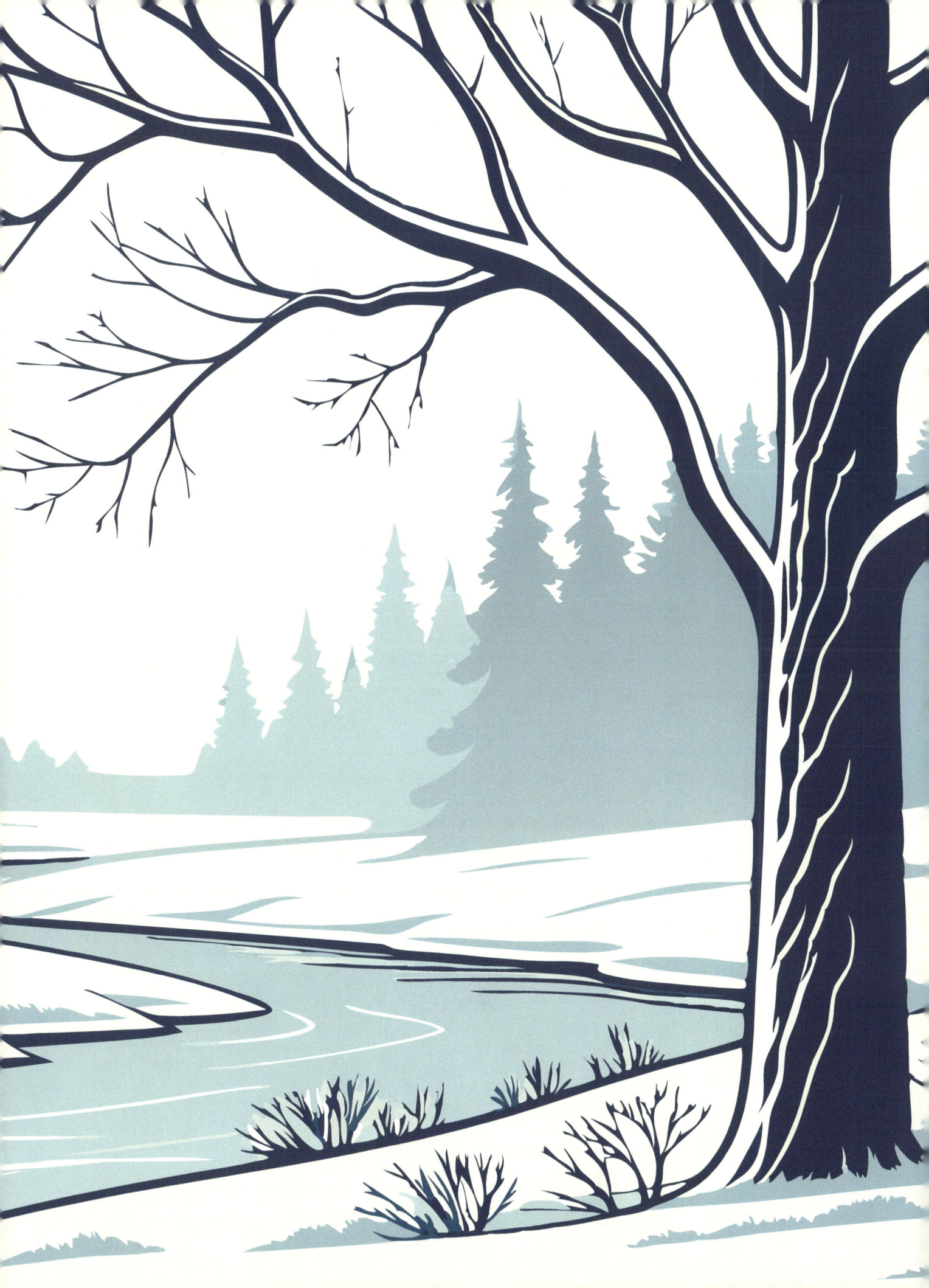

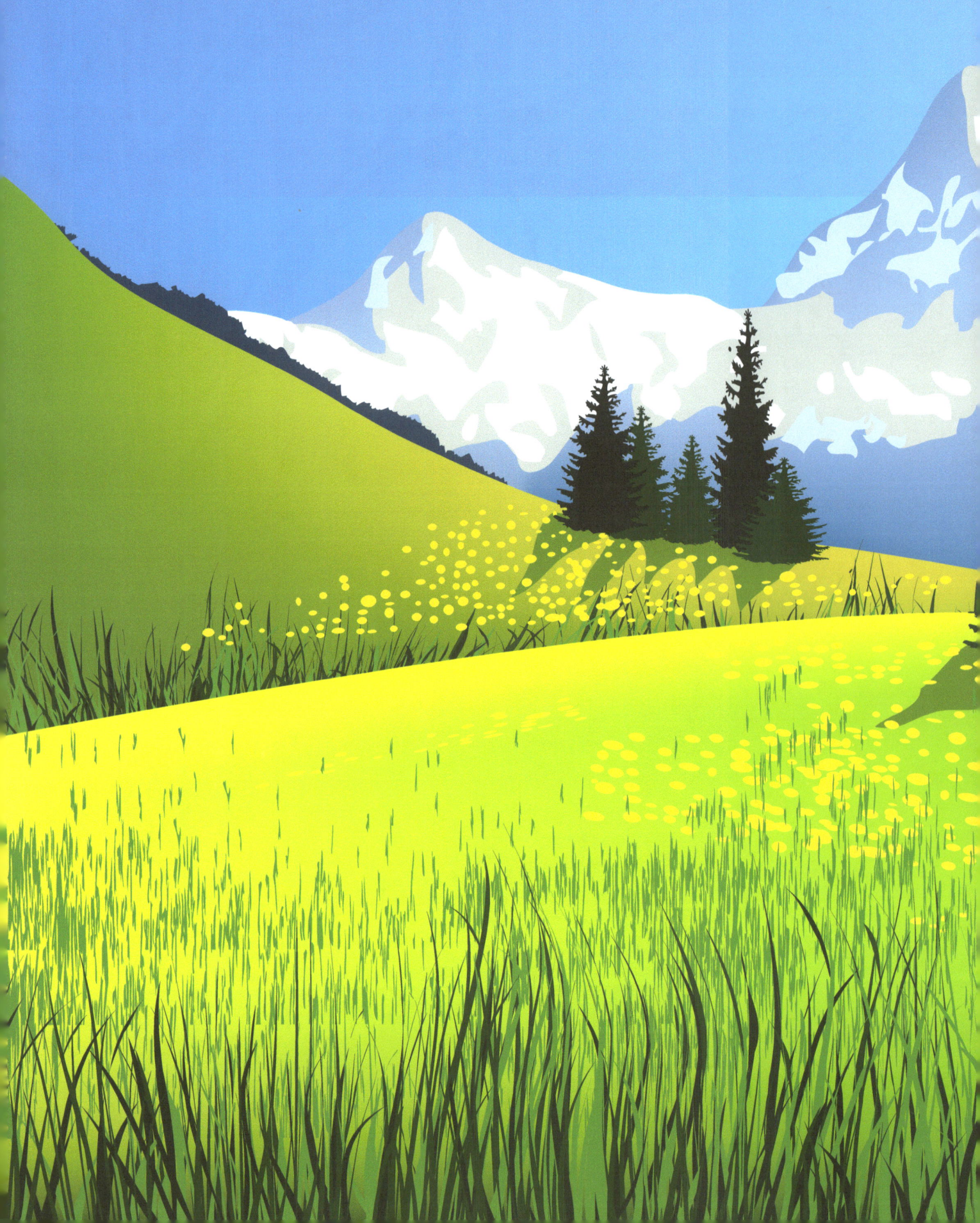

Grasslands and Meadows

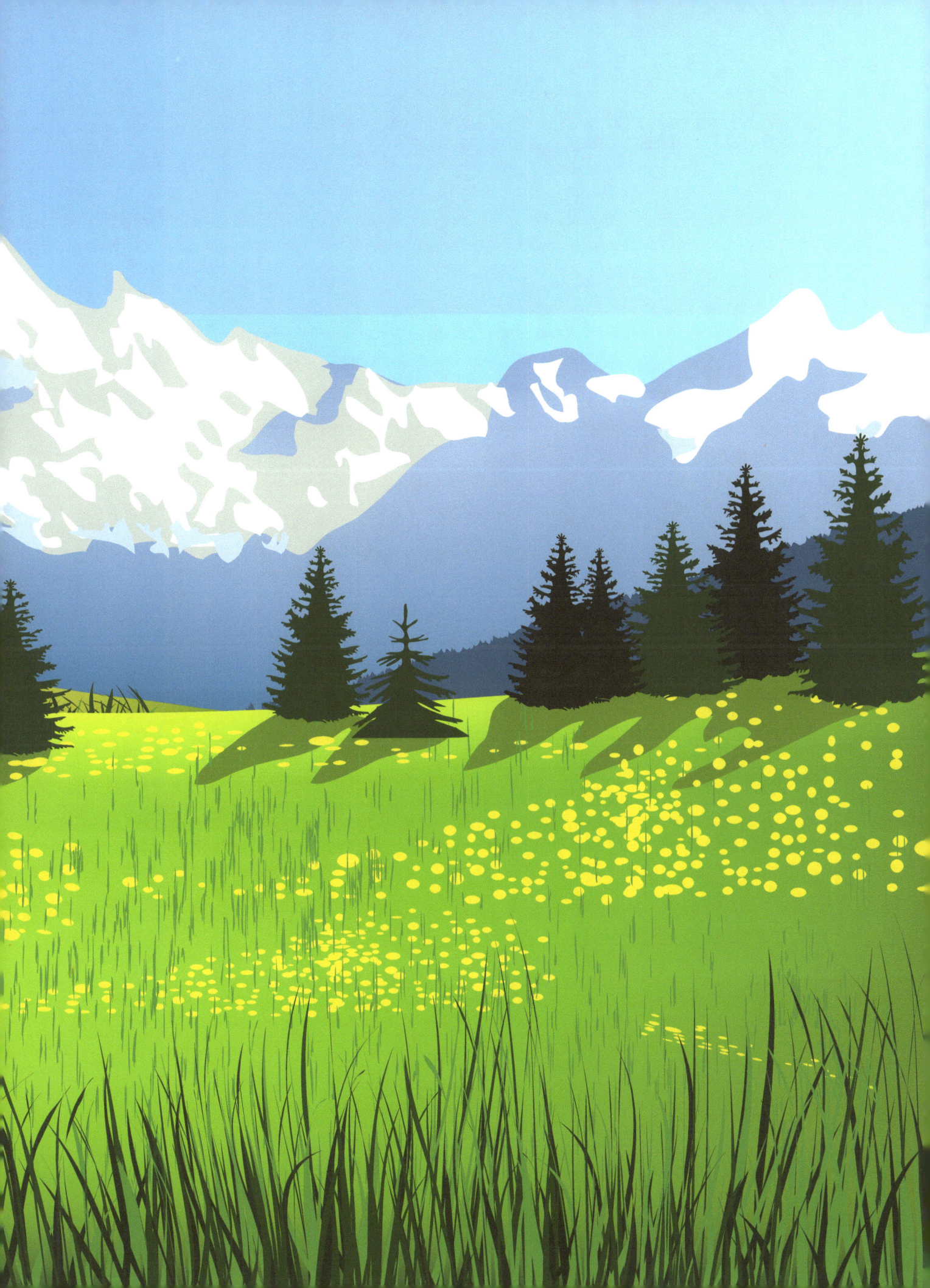

Lakes, Ponds, and Freshwater Wetlands

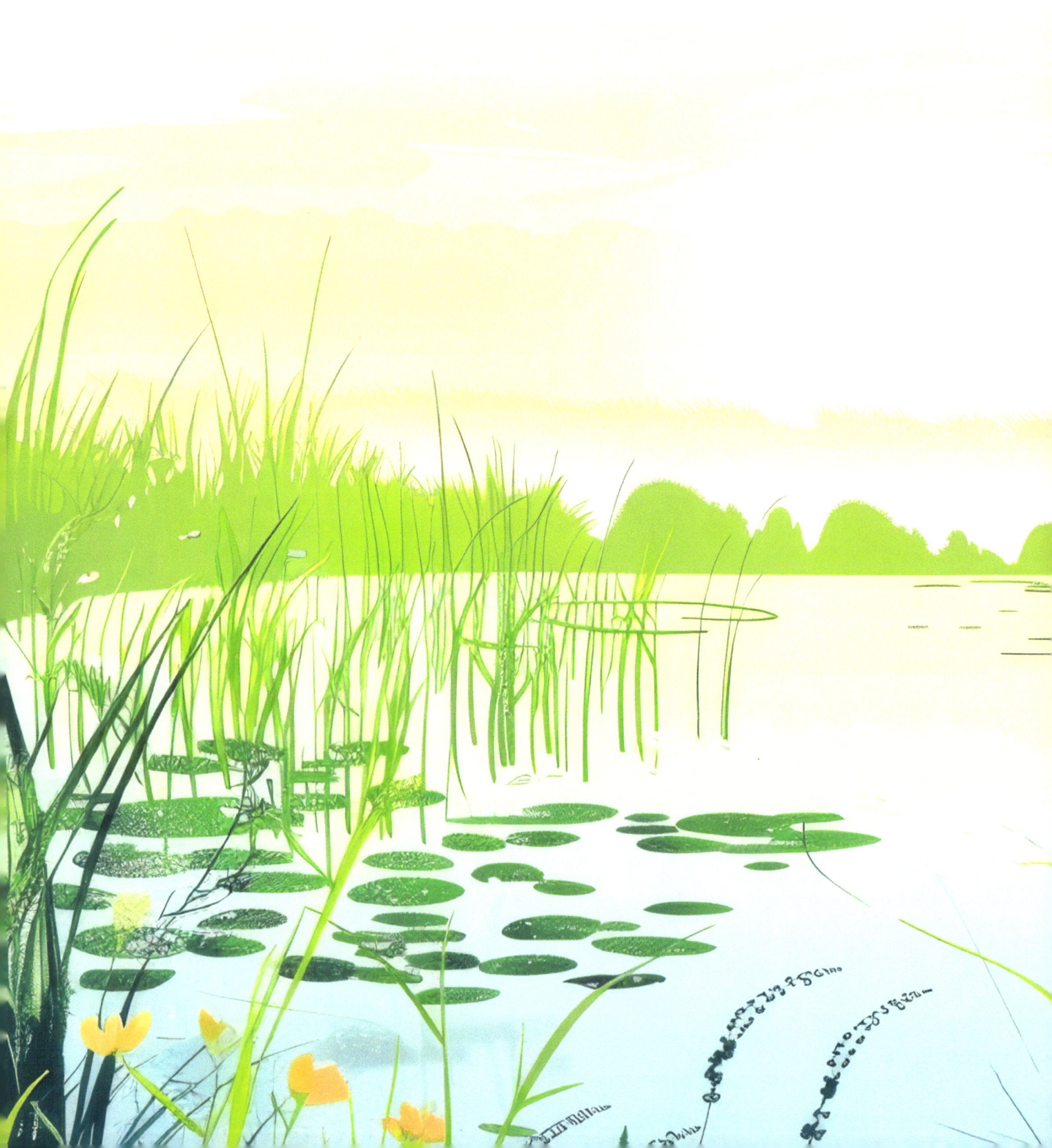

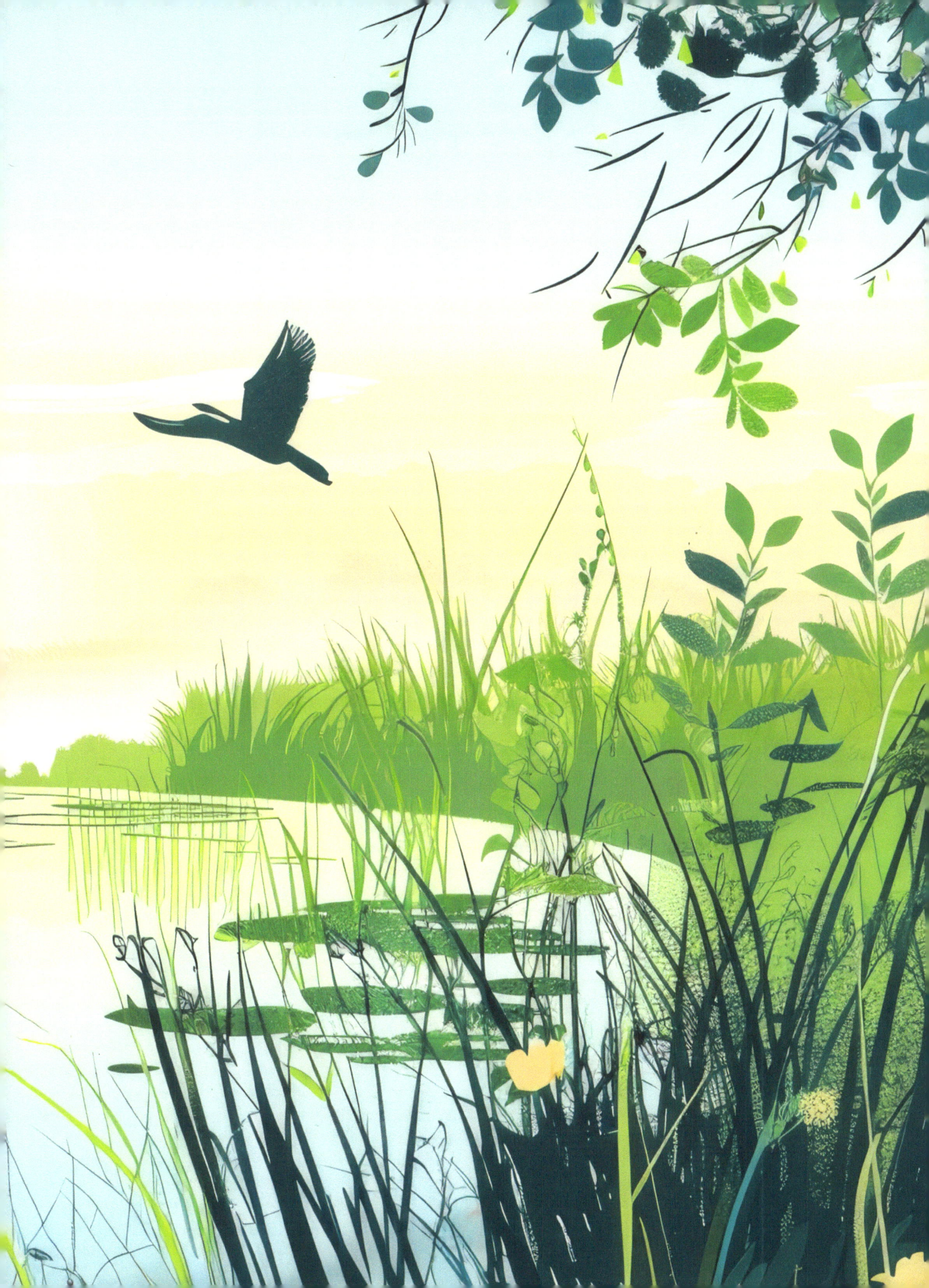

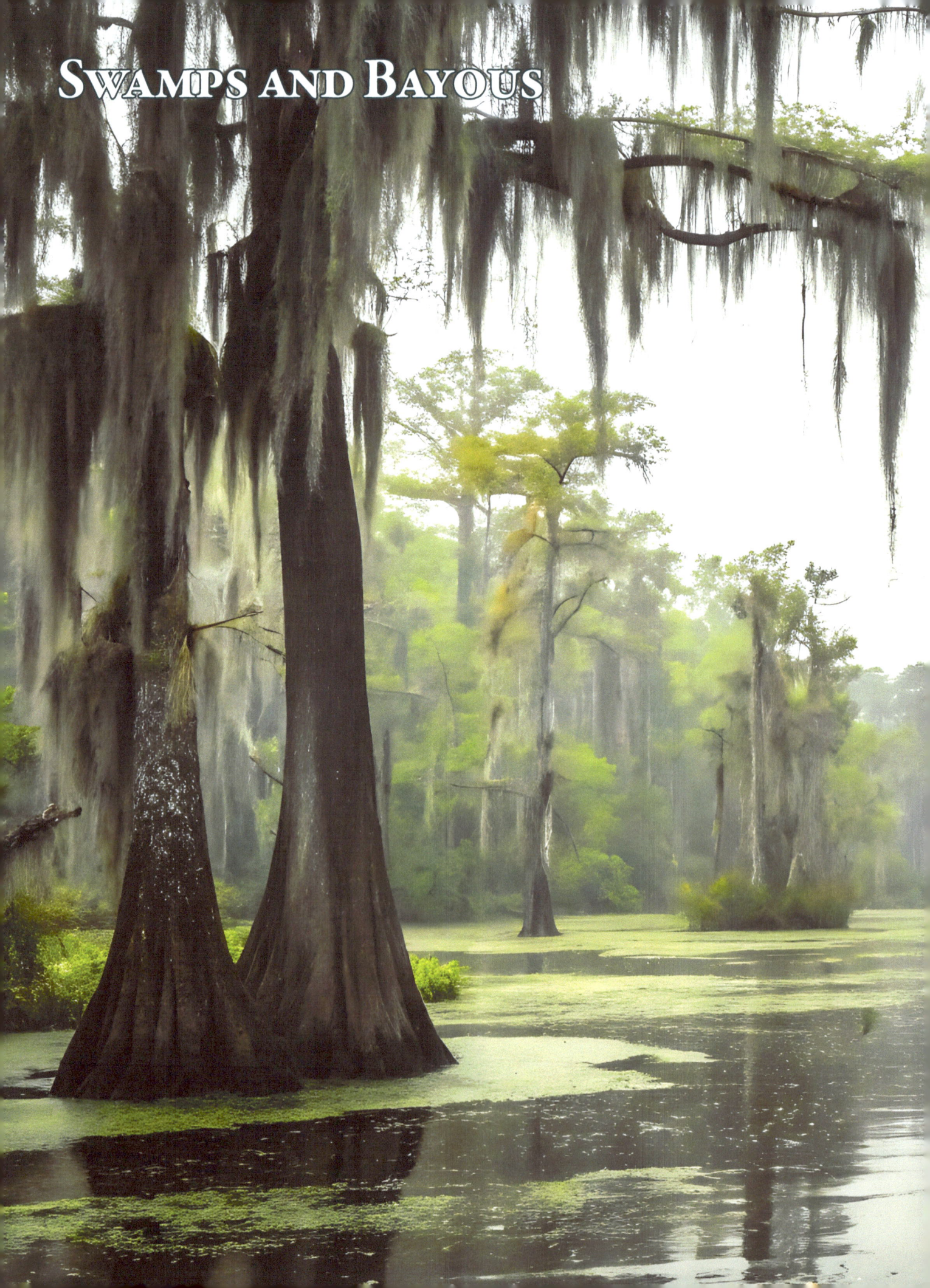

Swamps and Bayous

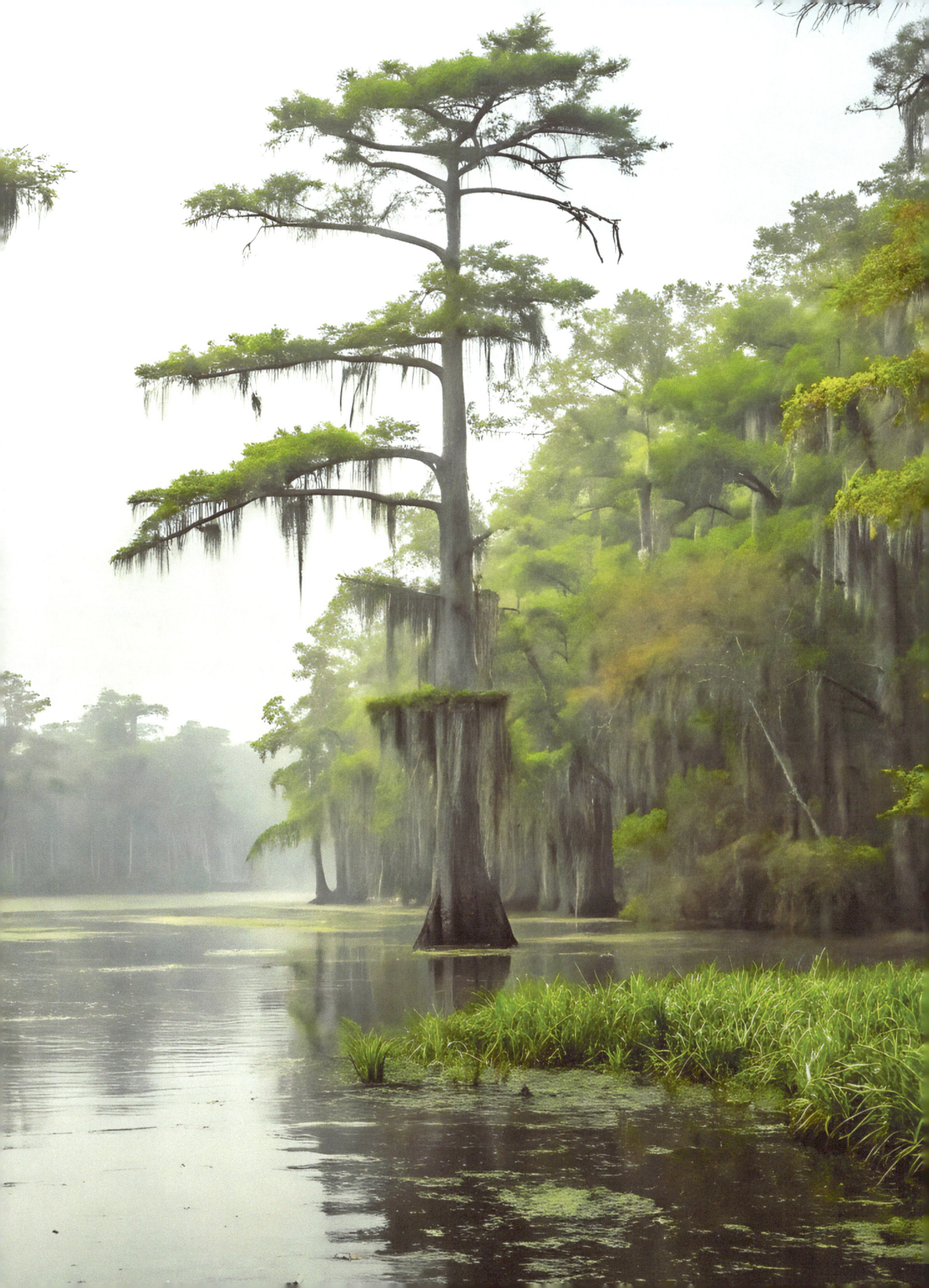

Mangroves

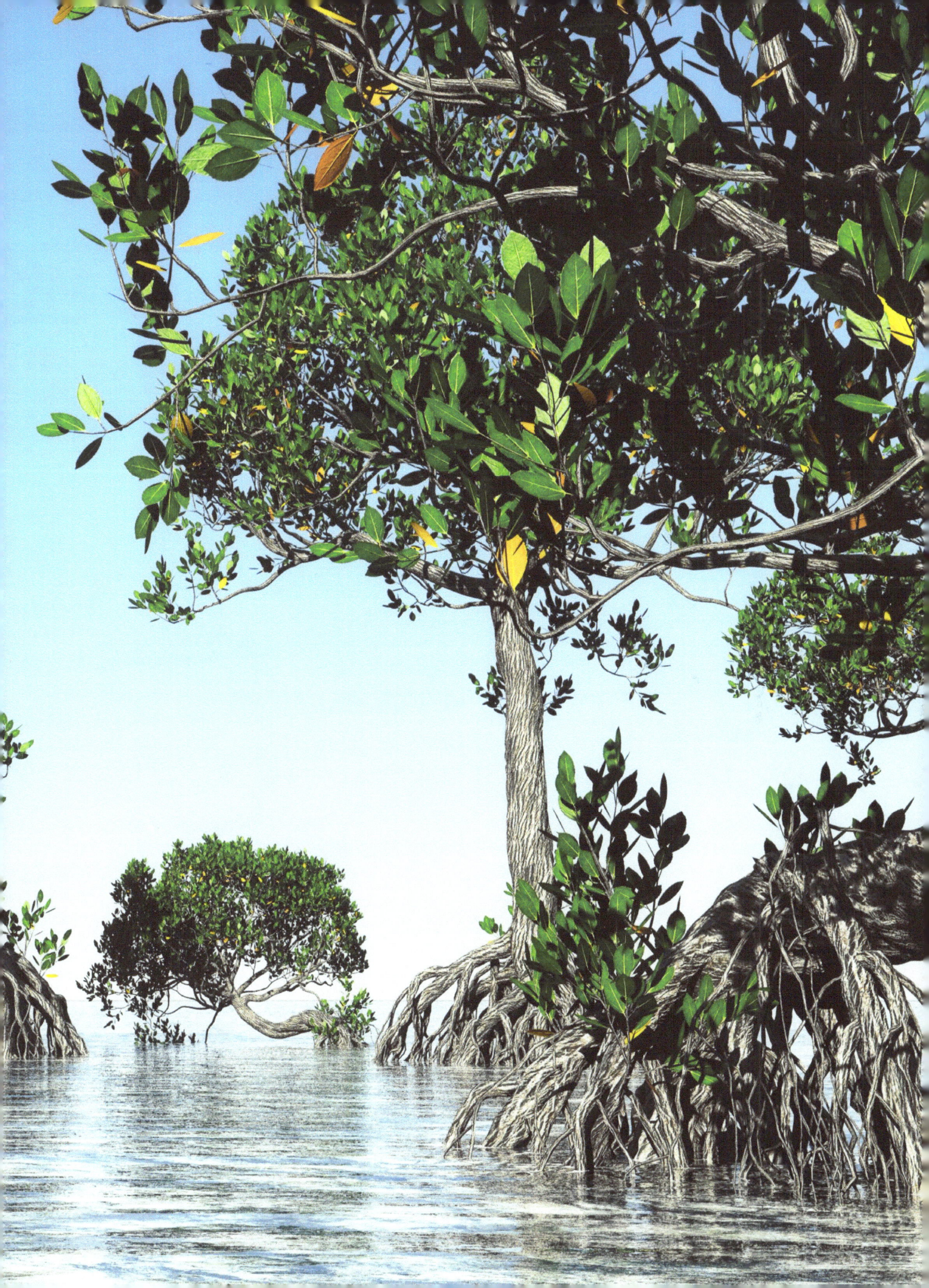

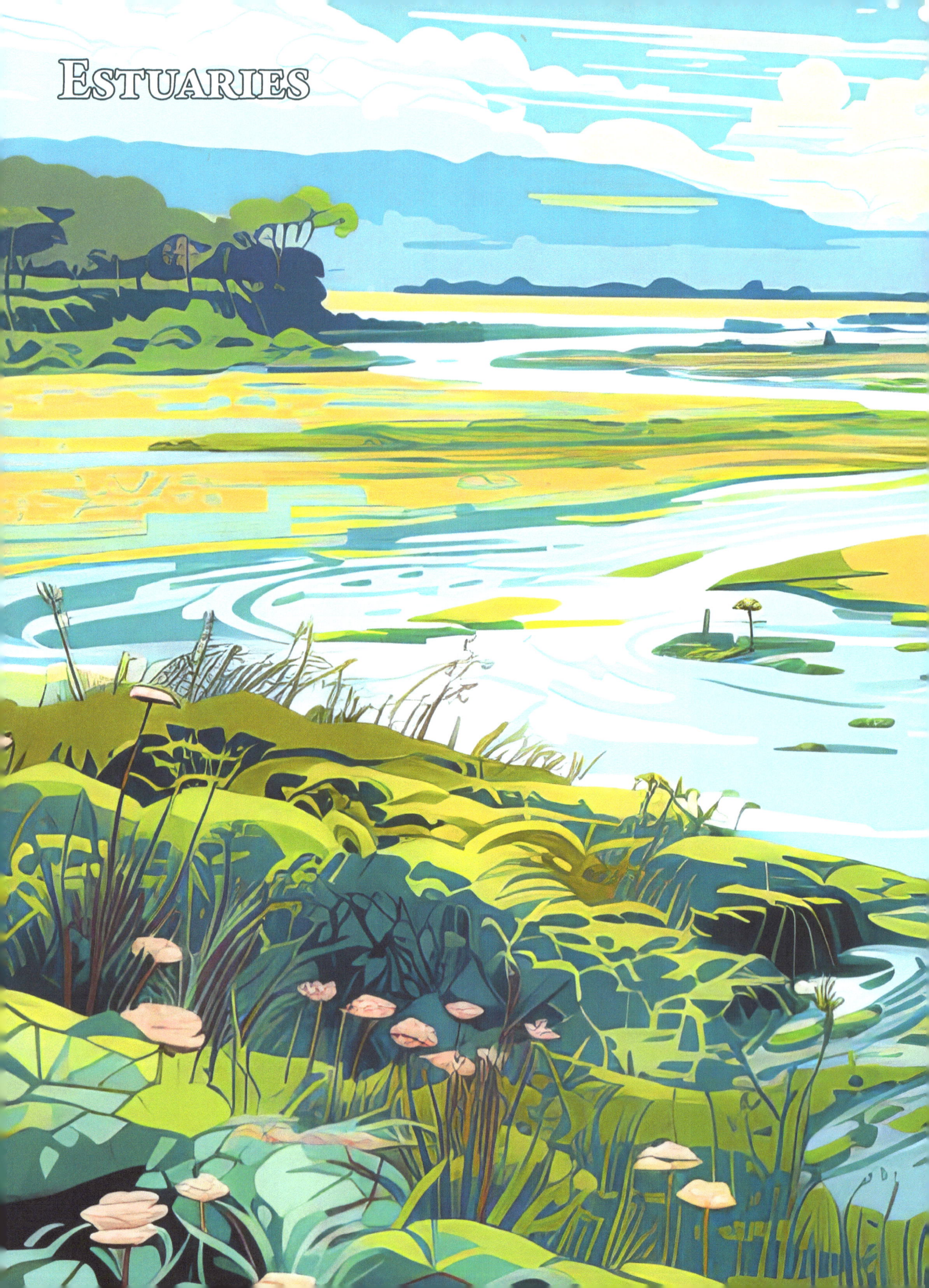

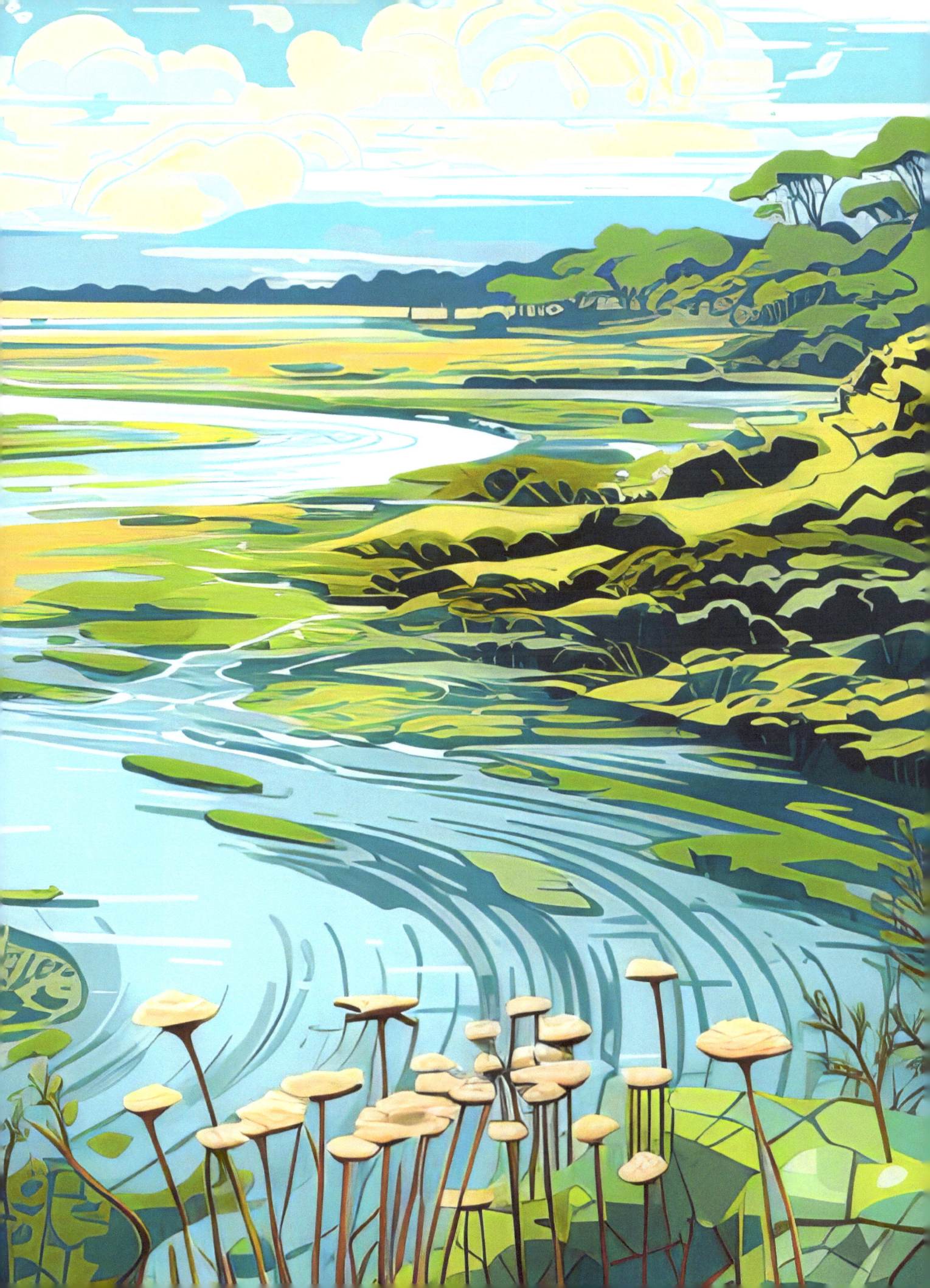

Sand Dunes and Coastal Waters

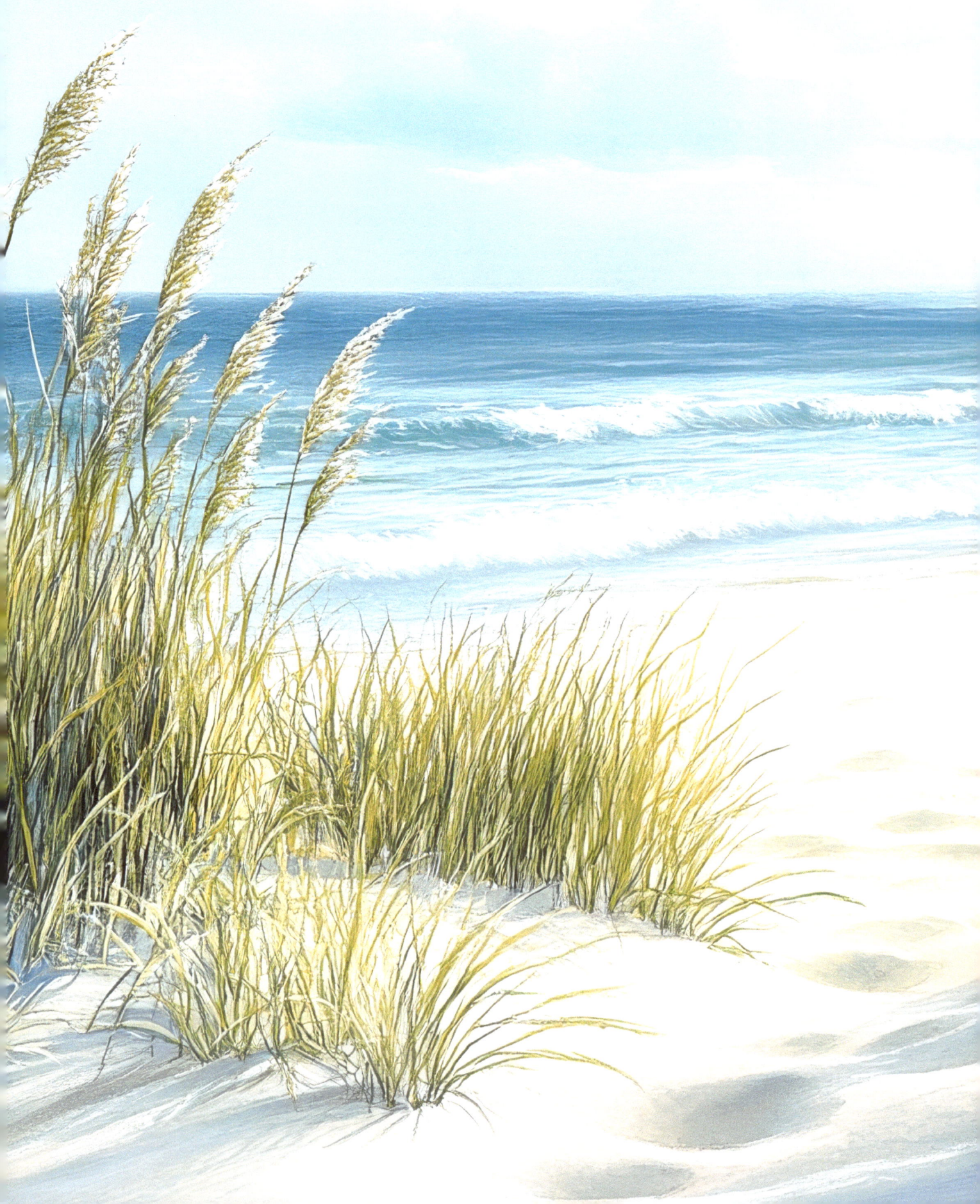

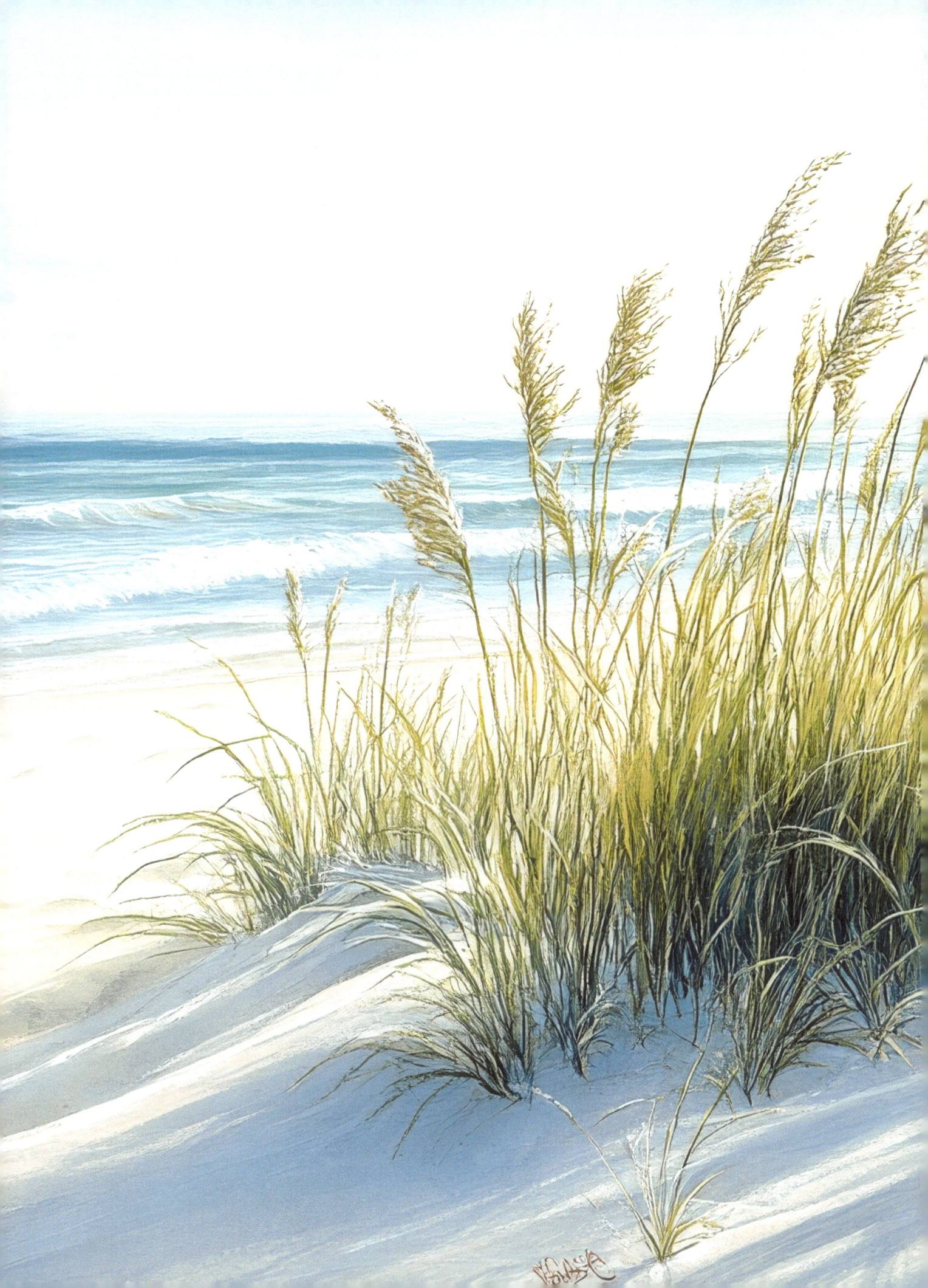

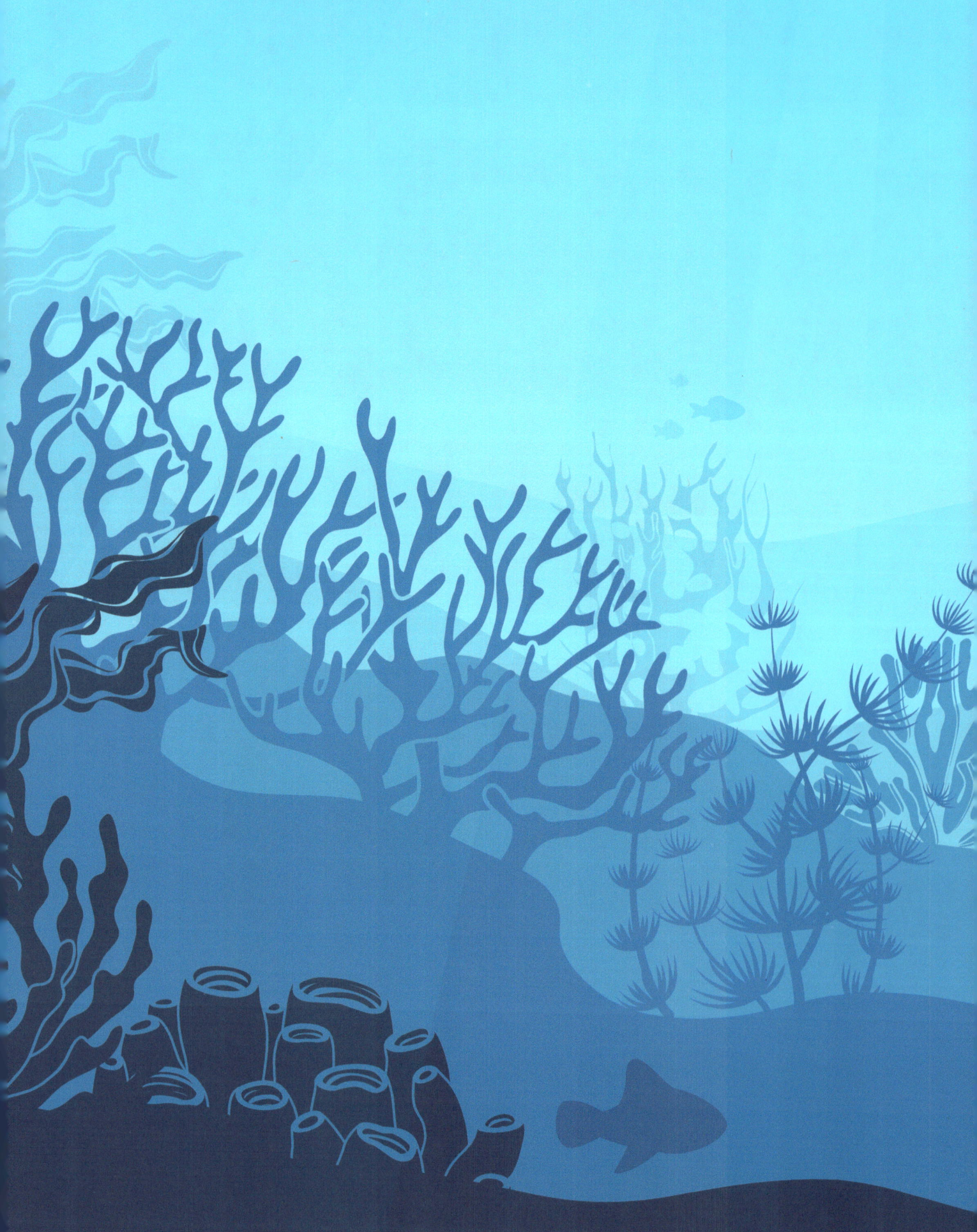

Coast and Ocean Floor

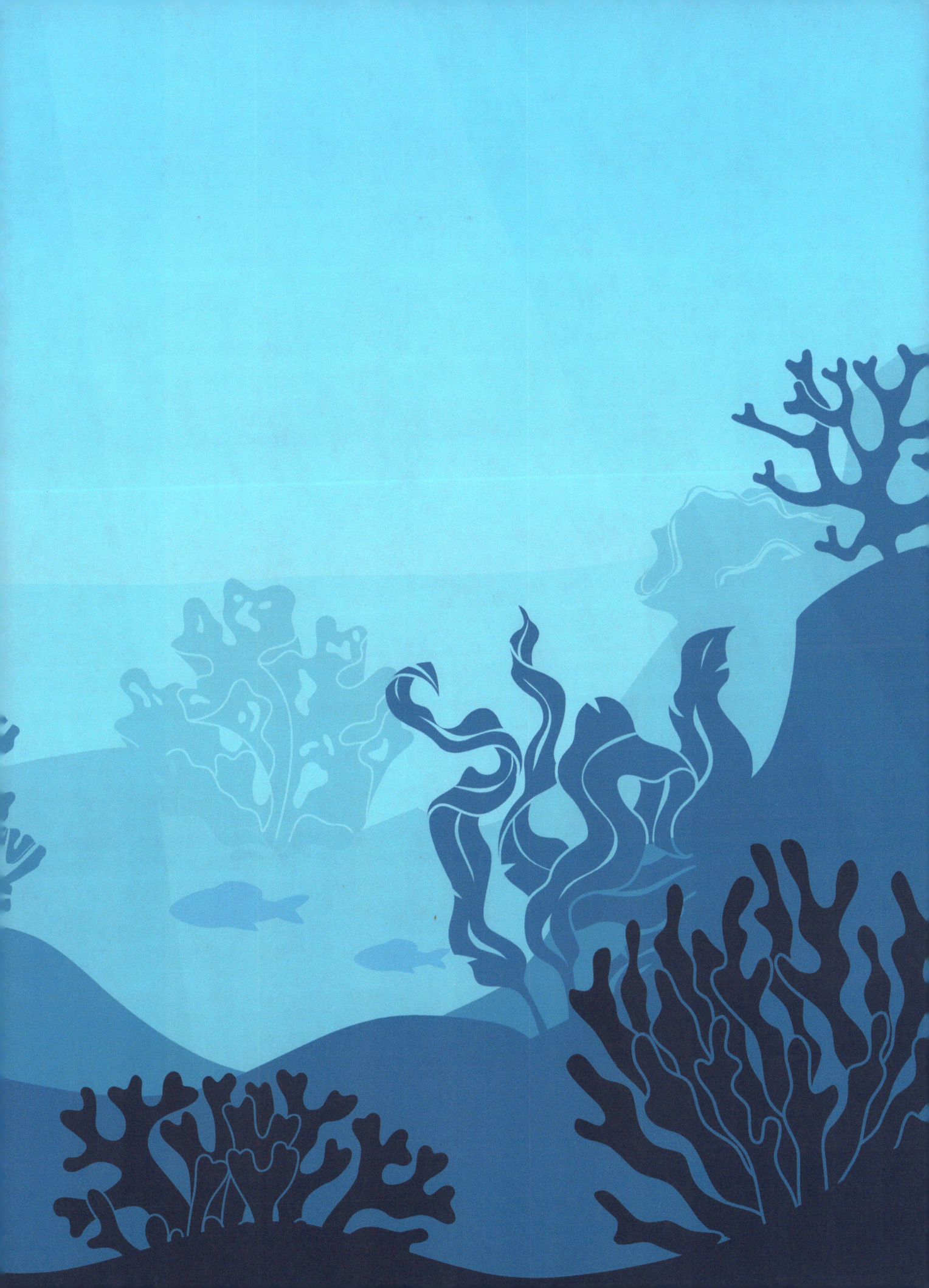

Deep Ocean

Deserts and Mountains

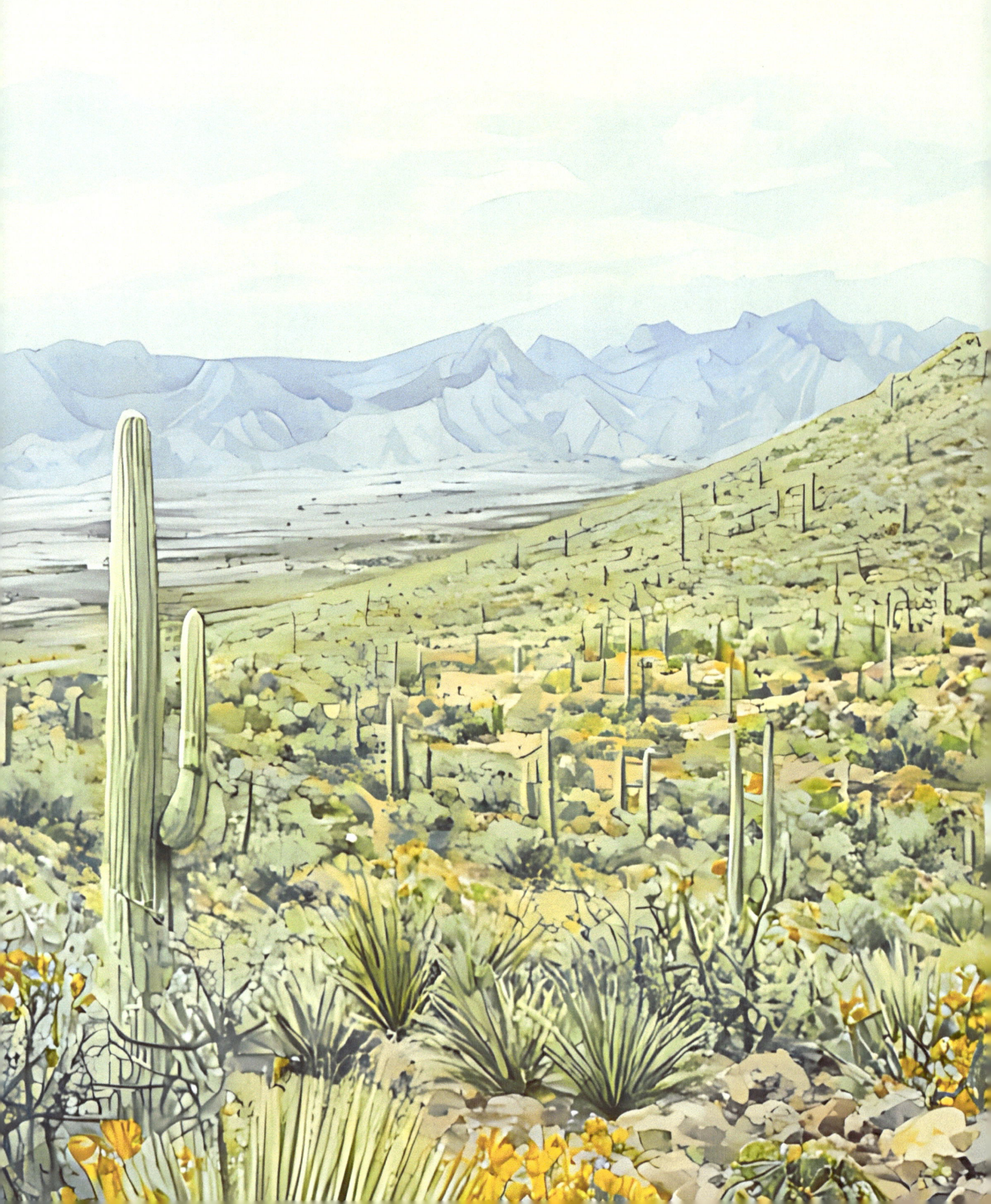

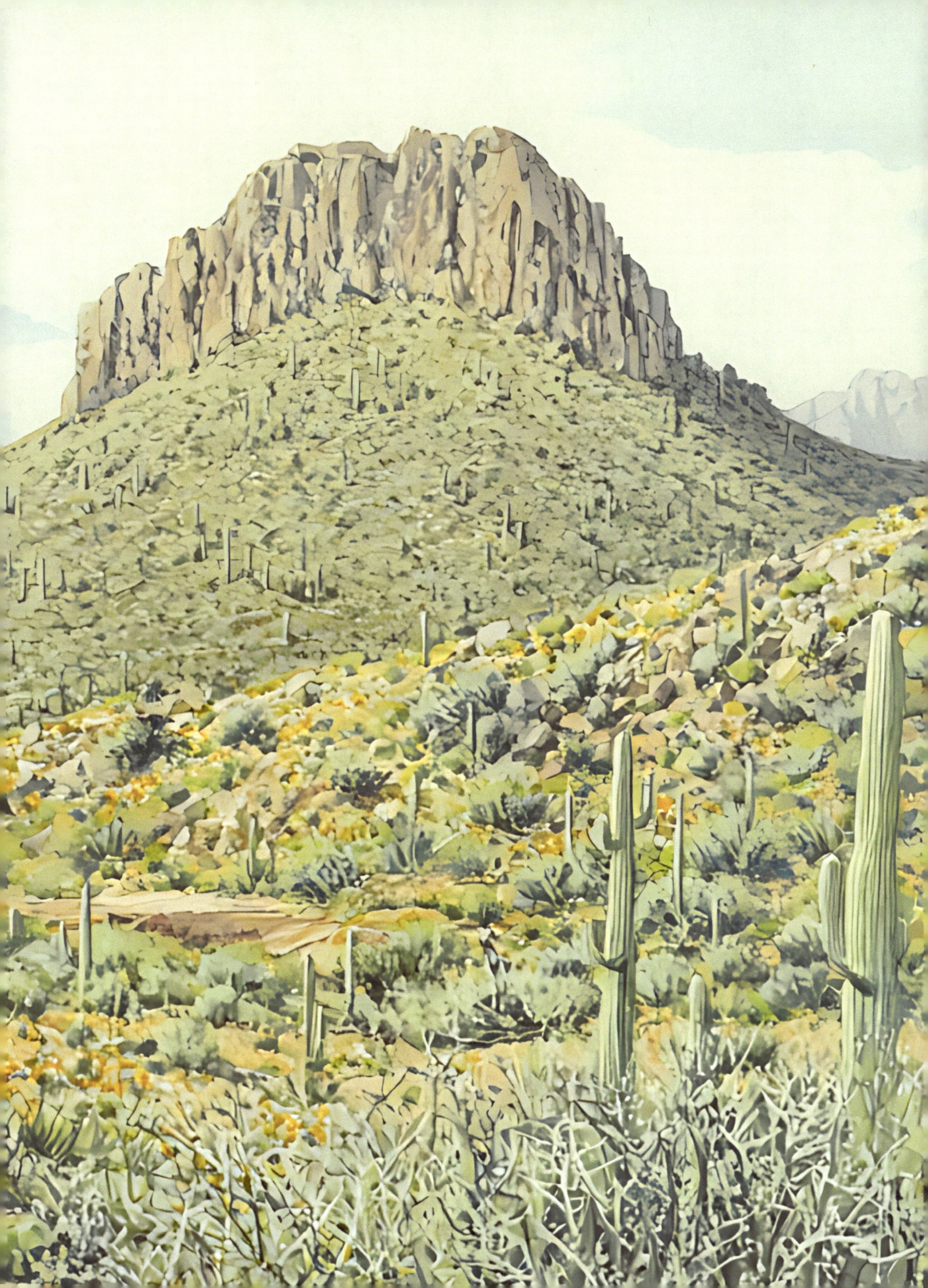

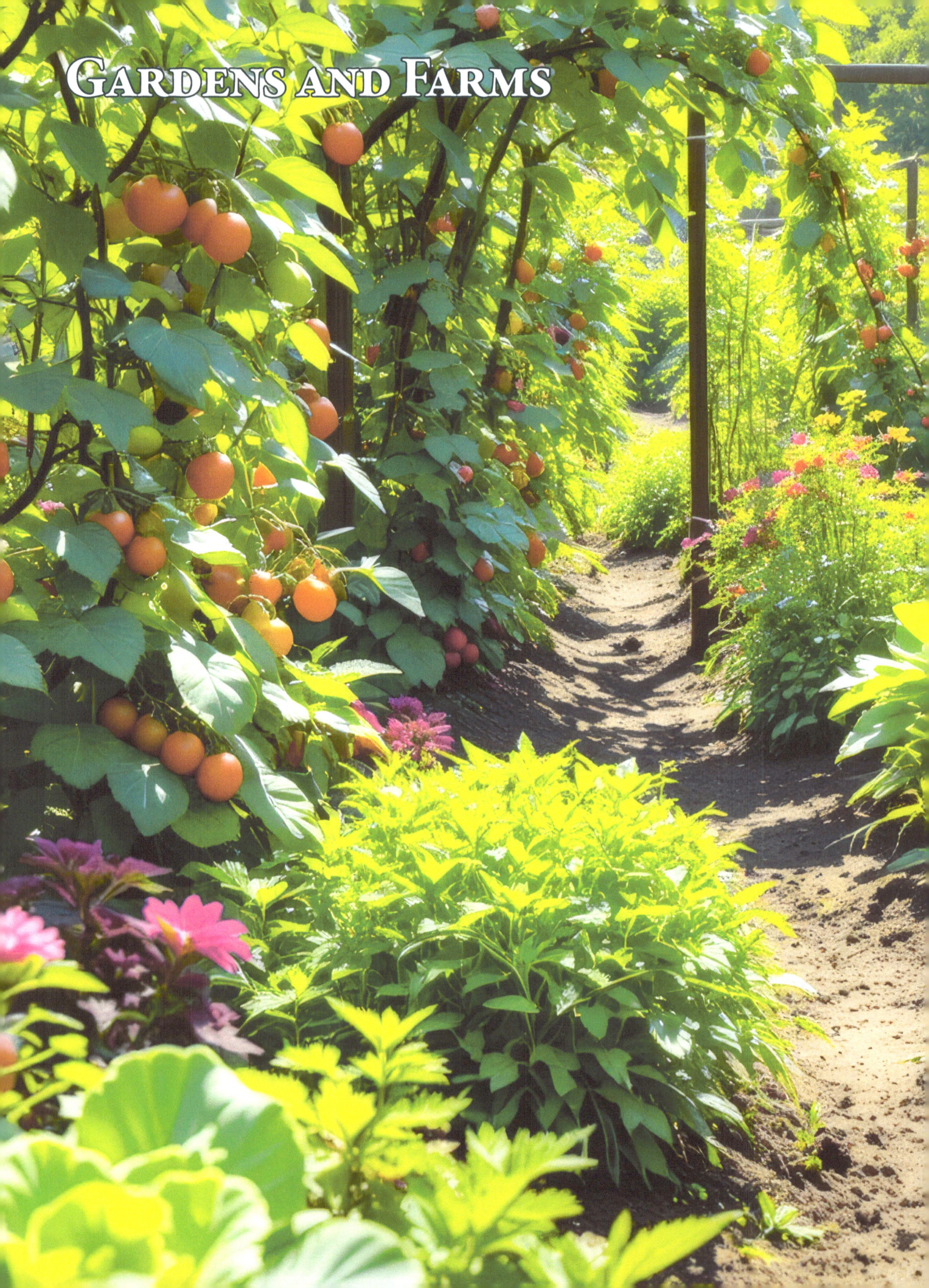
Gardens and Farms

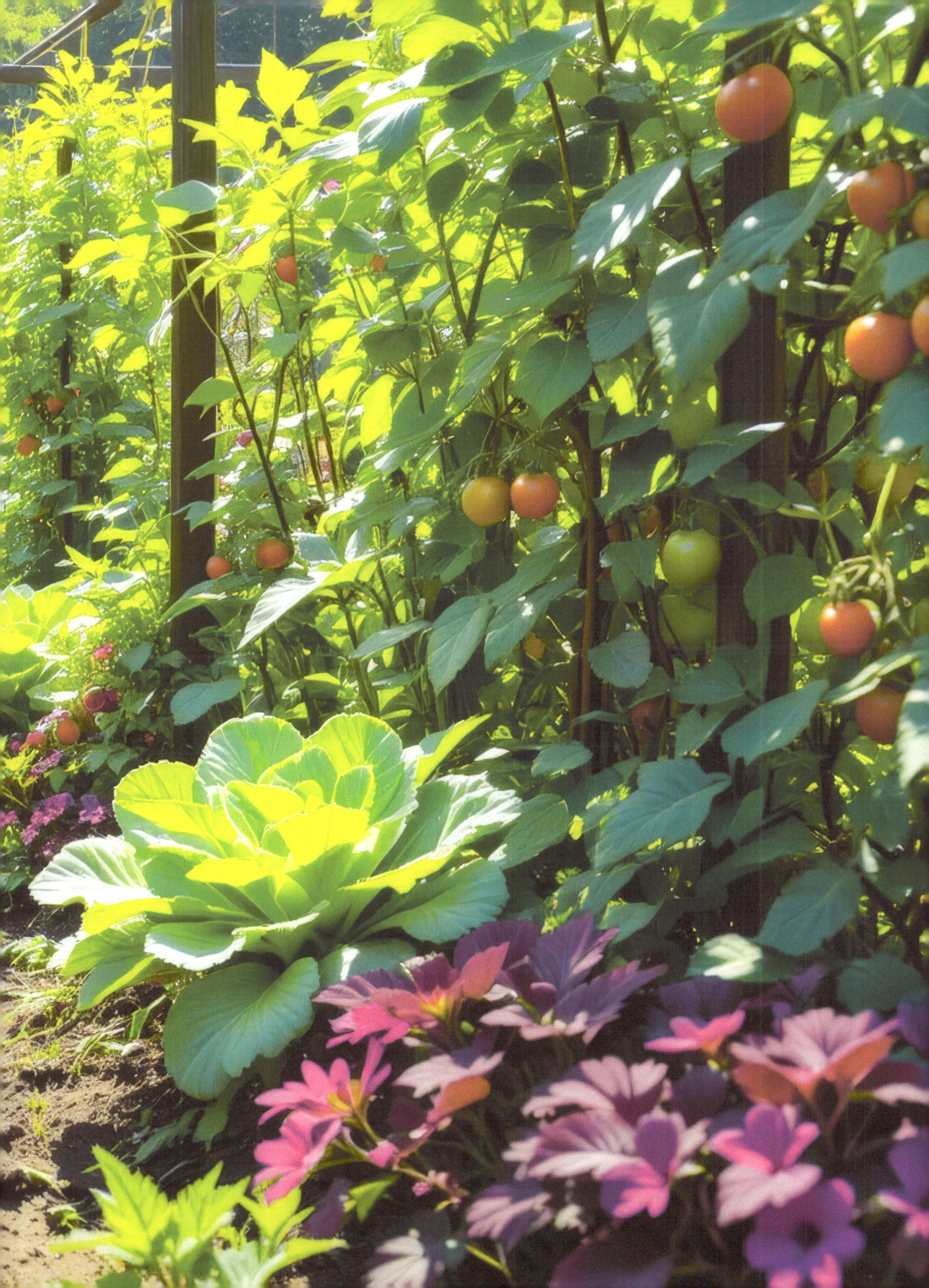

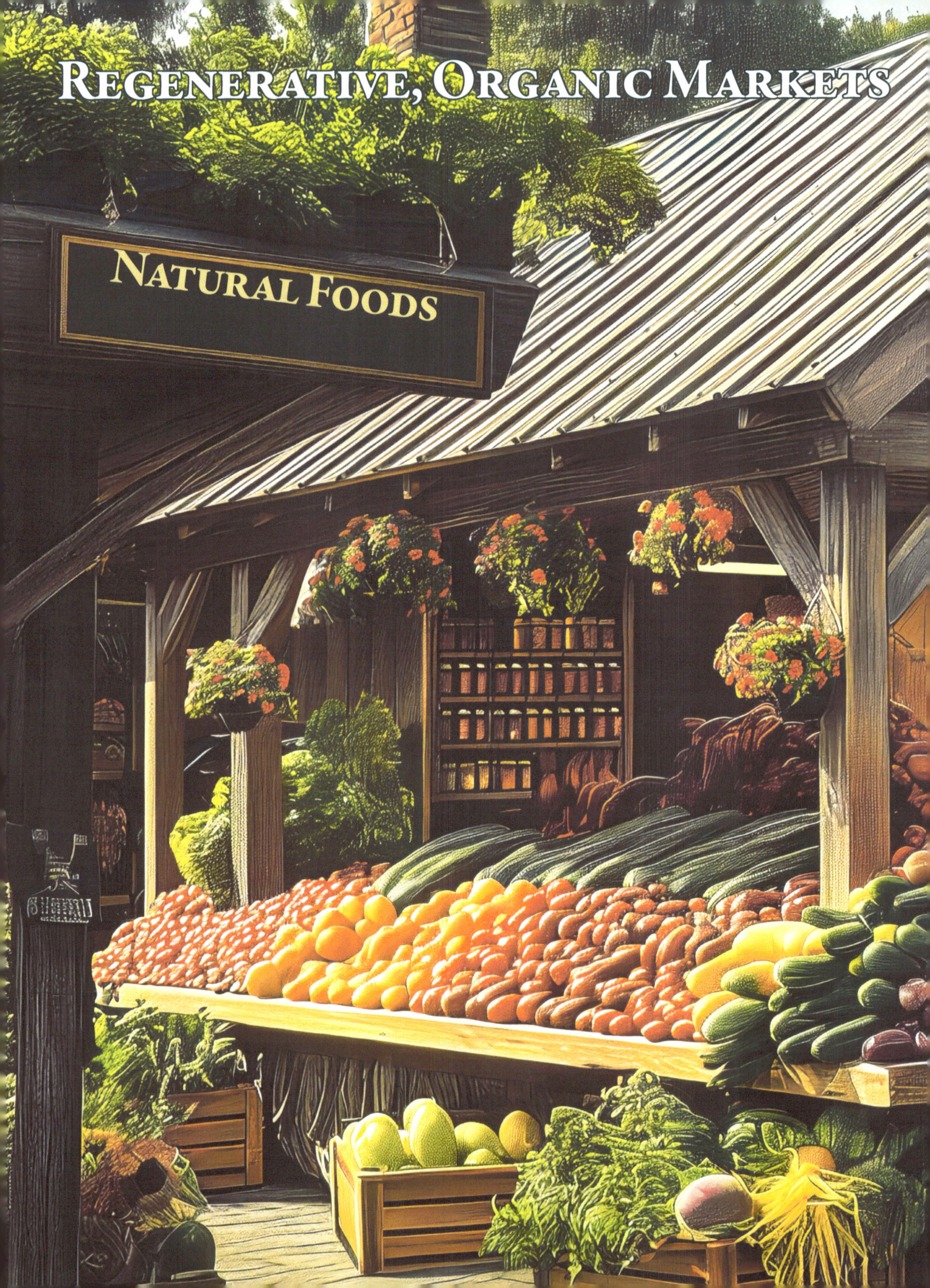

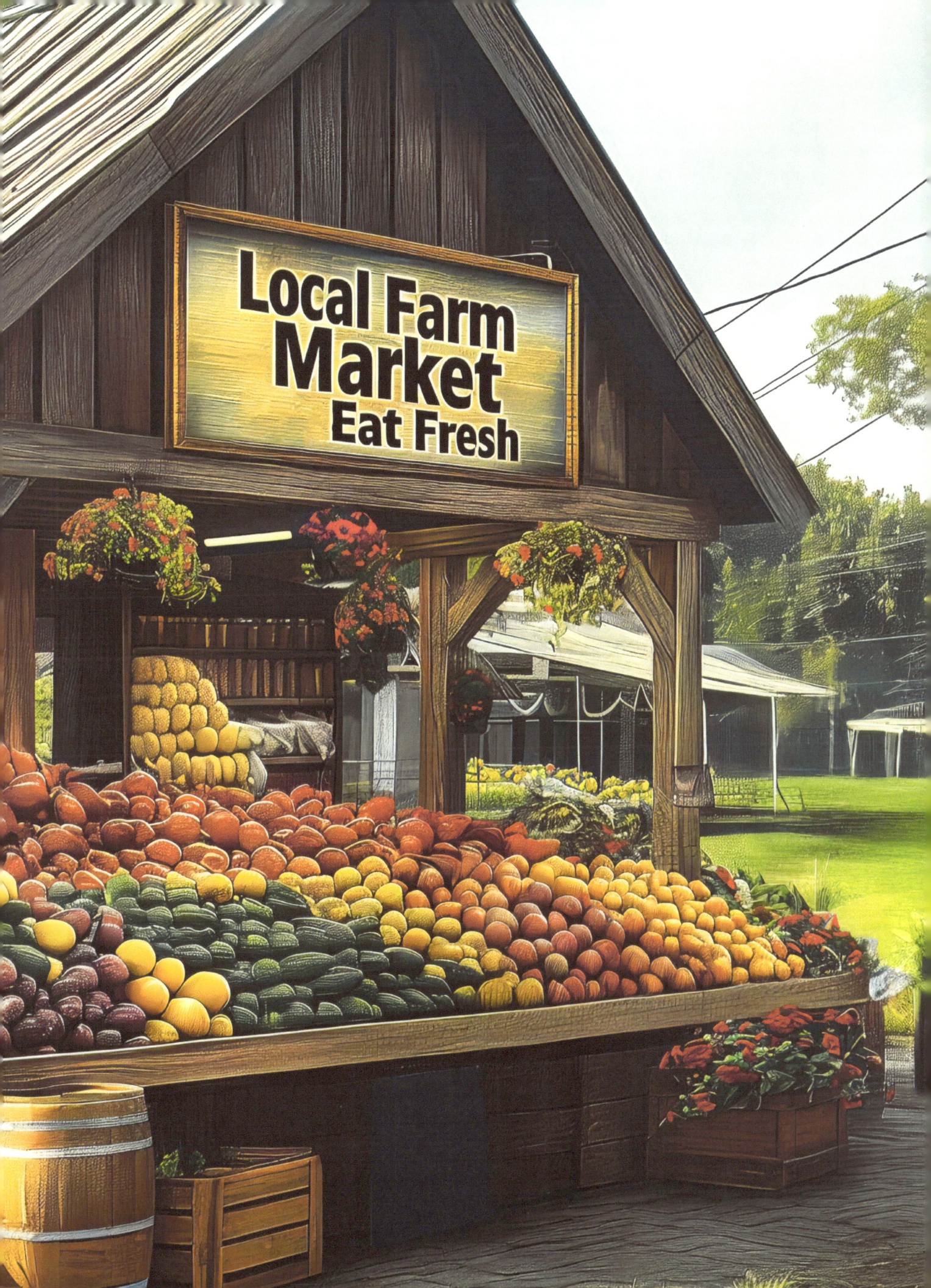

Natural Foods
from the Tapestry *of* Life

Natural Foods Sticker Package Reference
(pages 66 - 89)

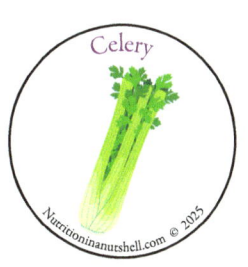
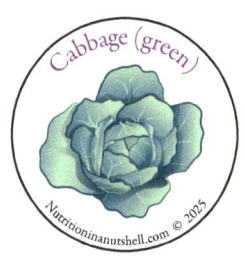
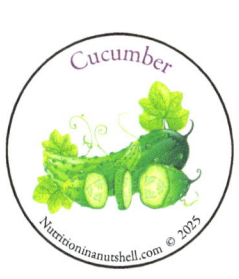
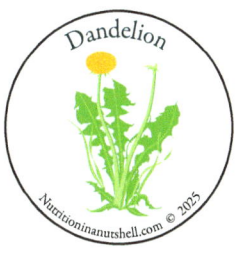
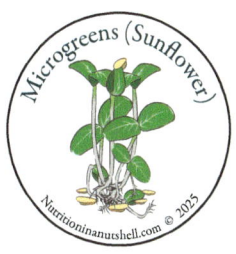

Seafoods

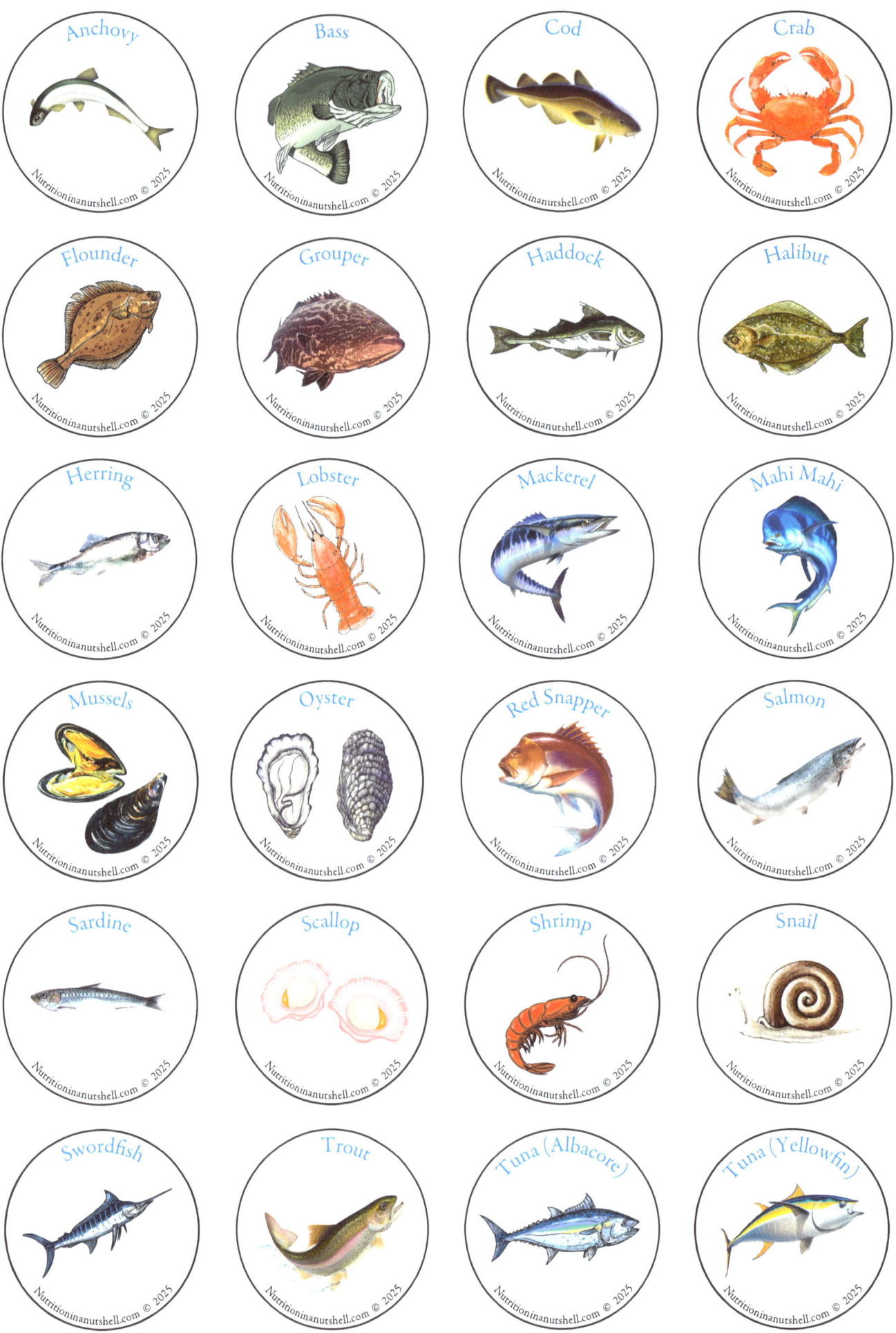

Seafoods

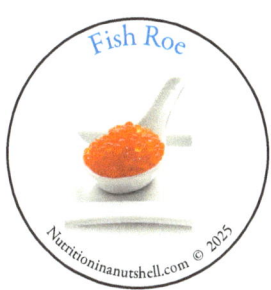 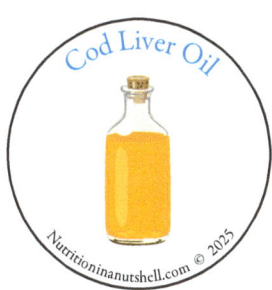 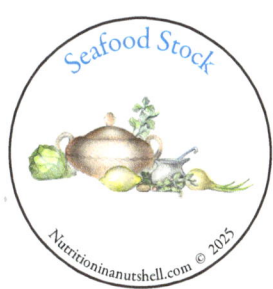 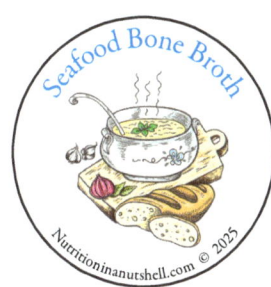

Meats

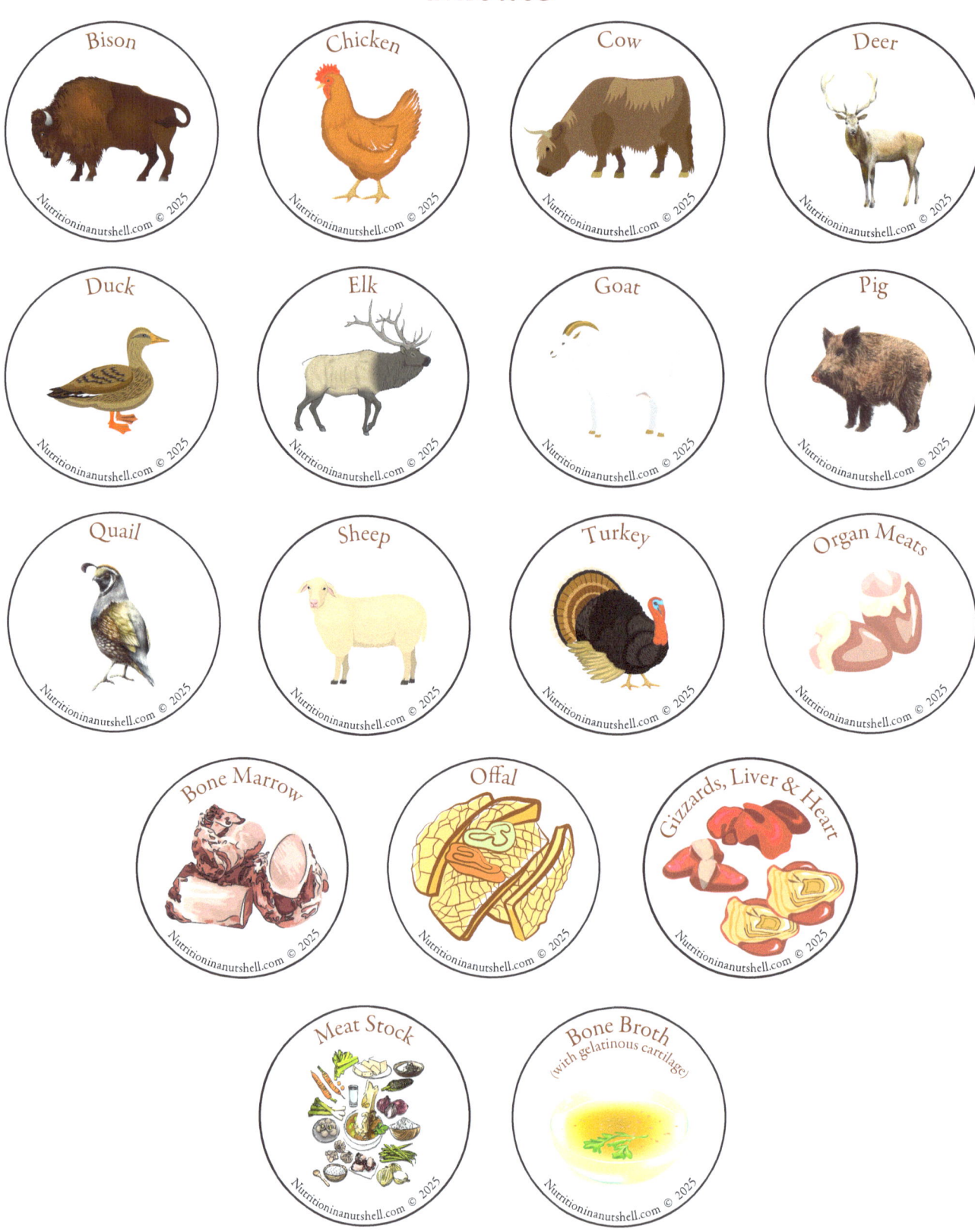

Milk Products

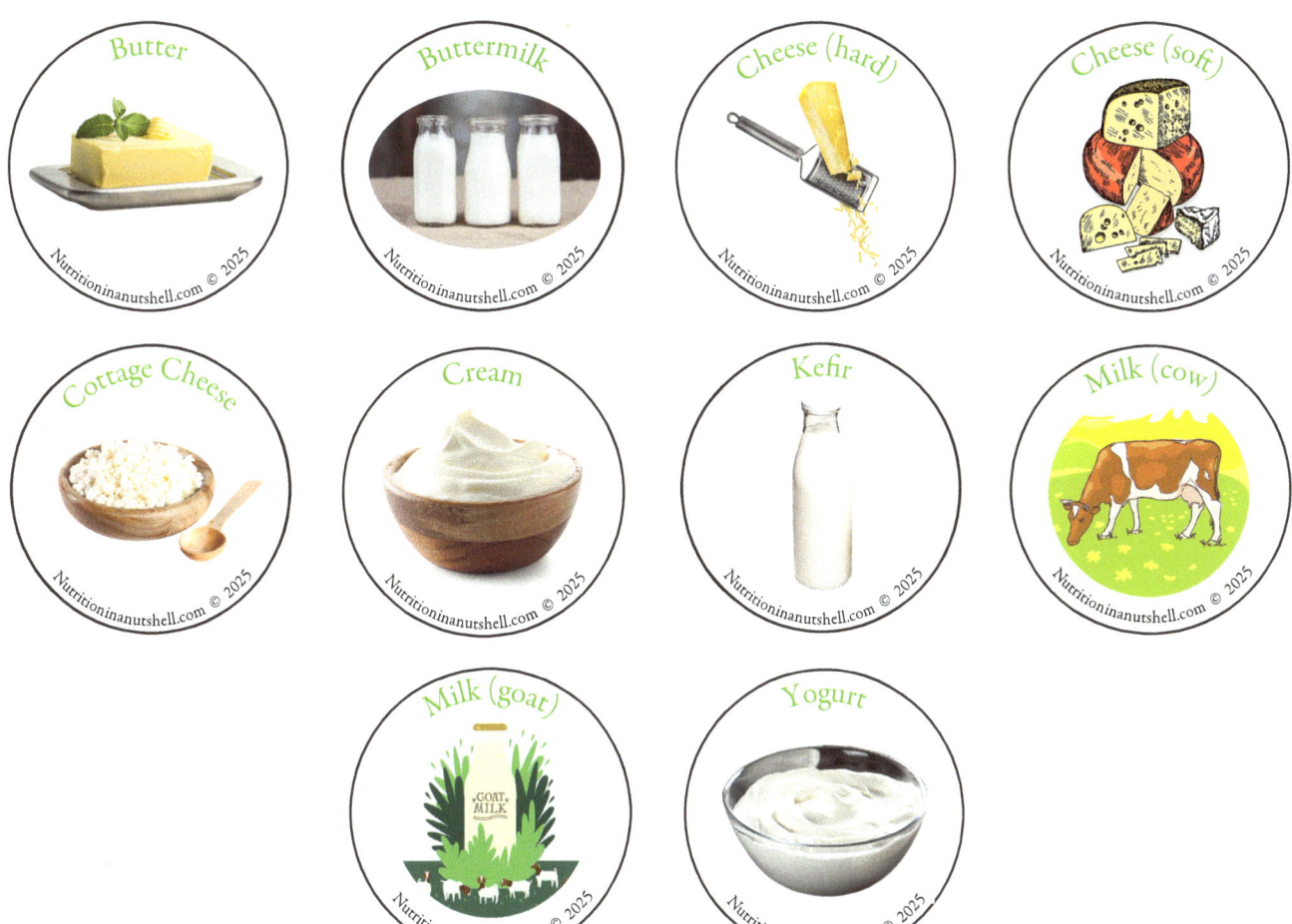

Land & Waterfowl Eggs

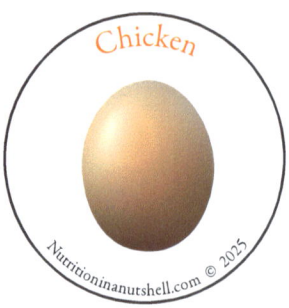 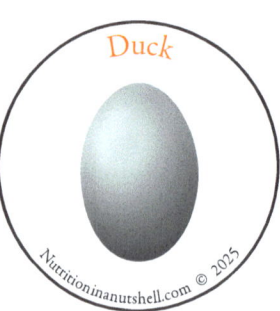 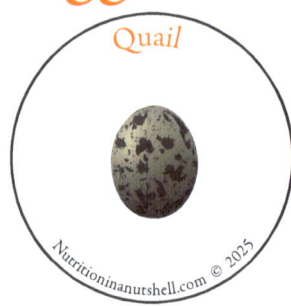

Chicken | Duck | Quail

Animal Fats

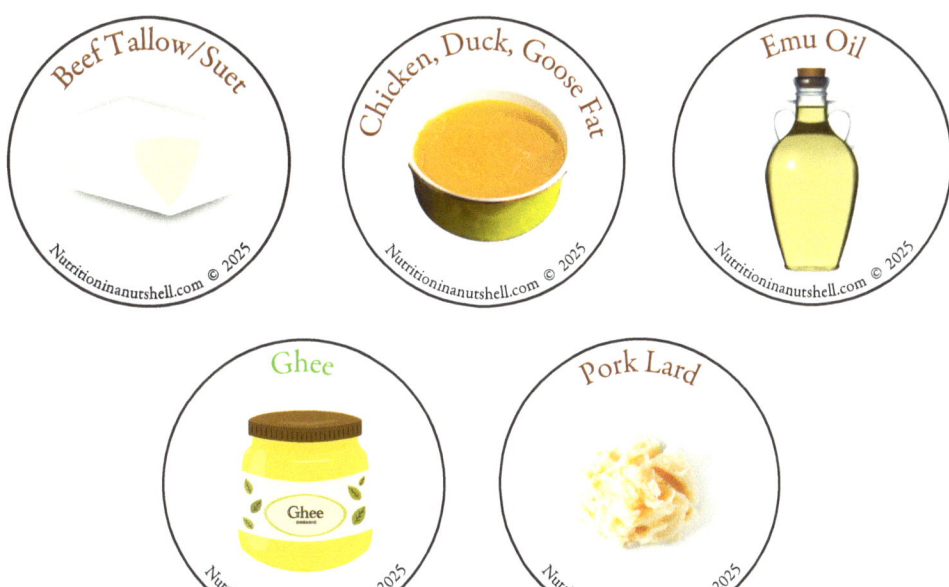

Fruits

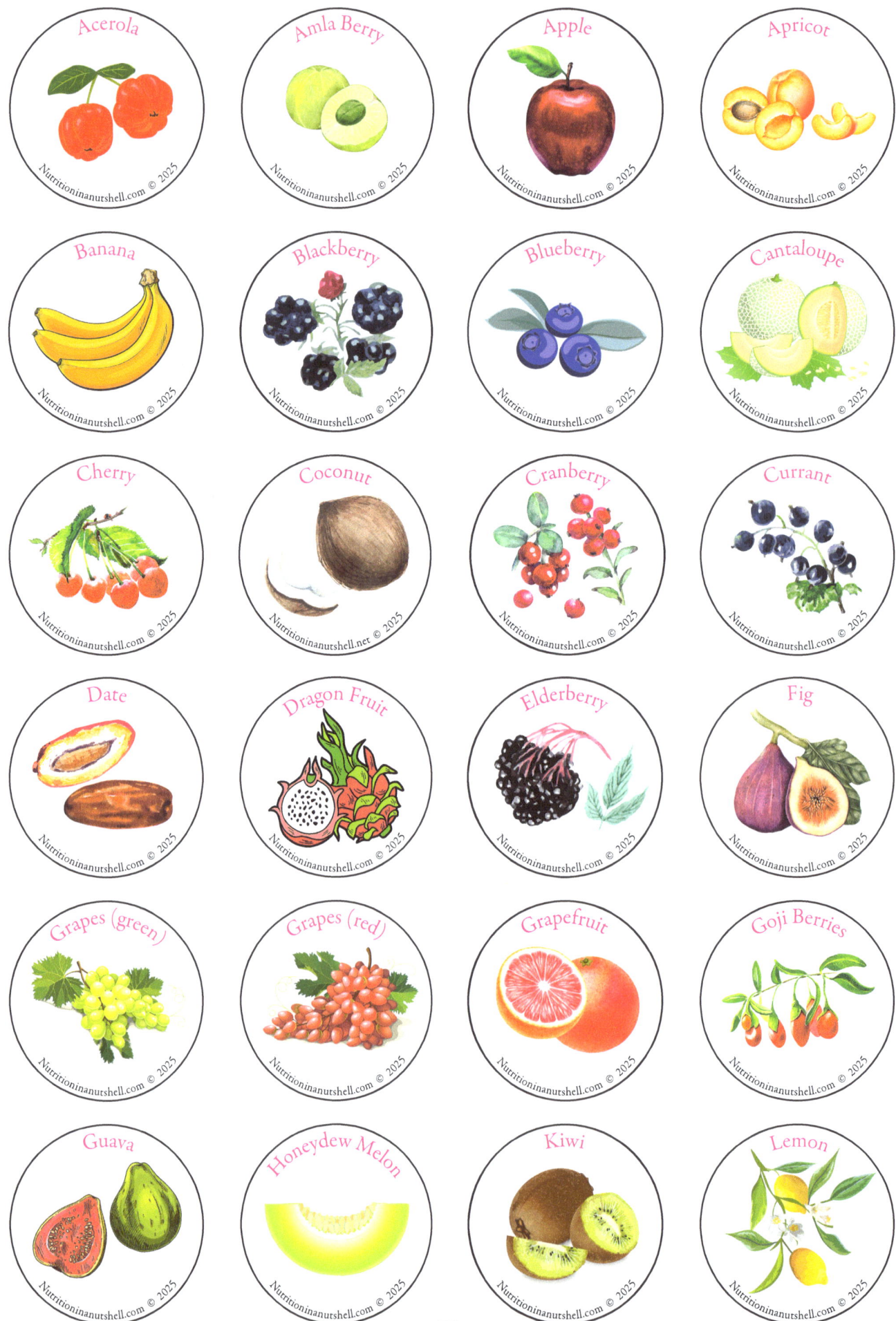

Fruits

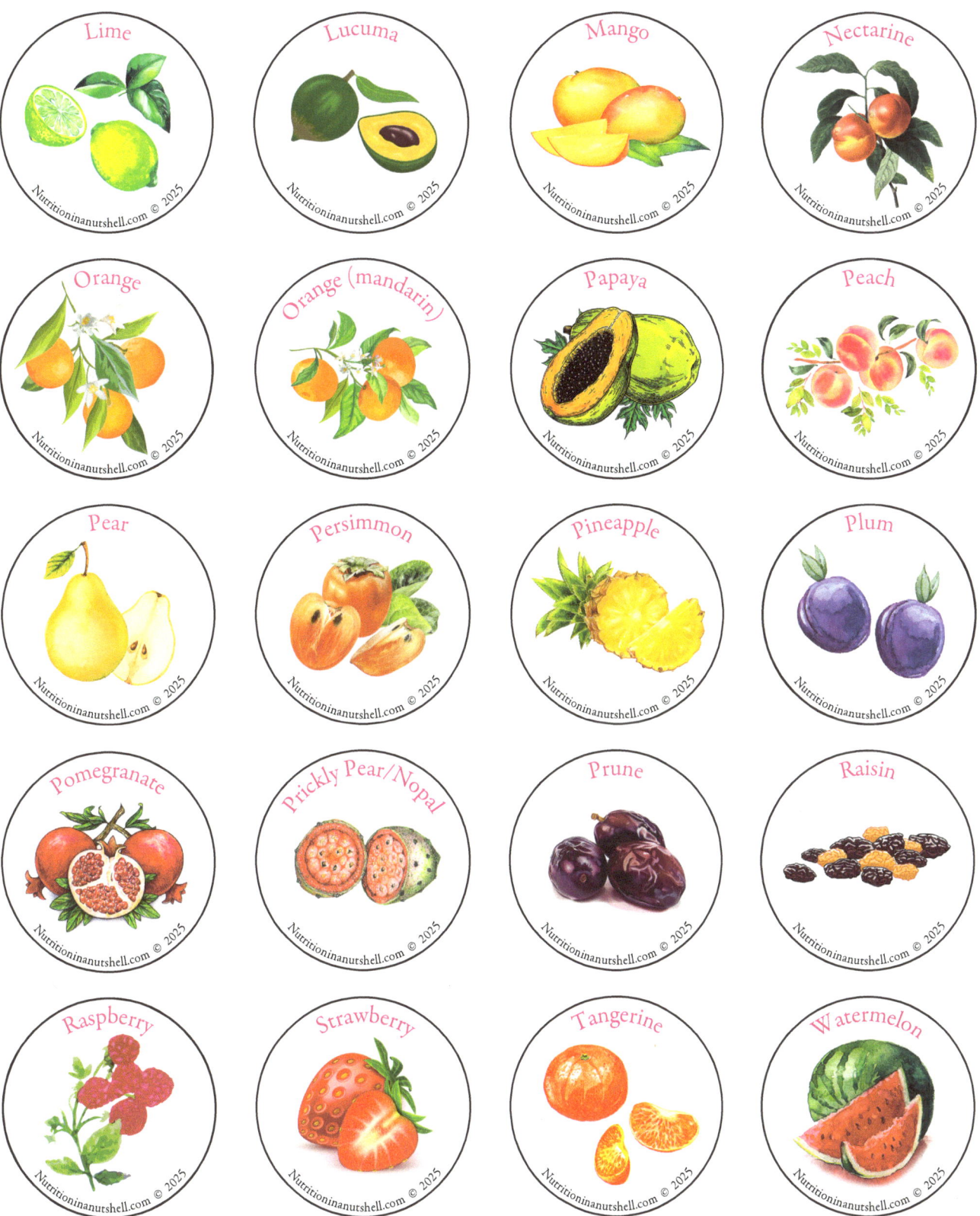

Grains

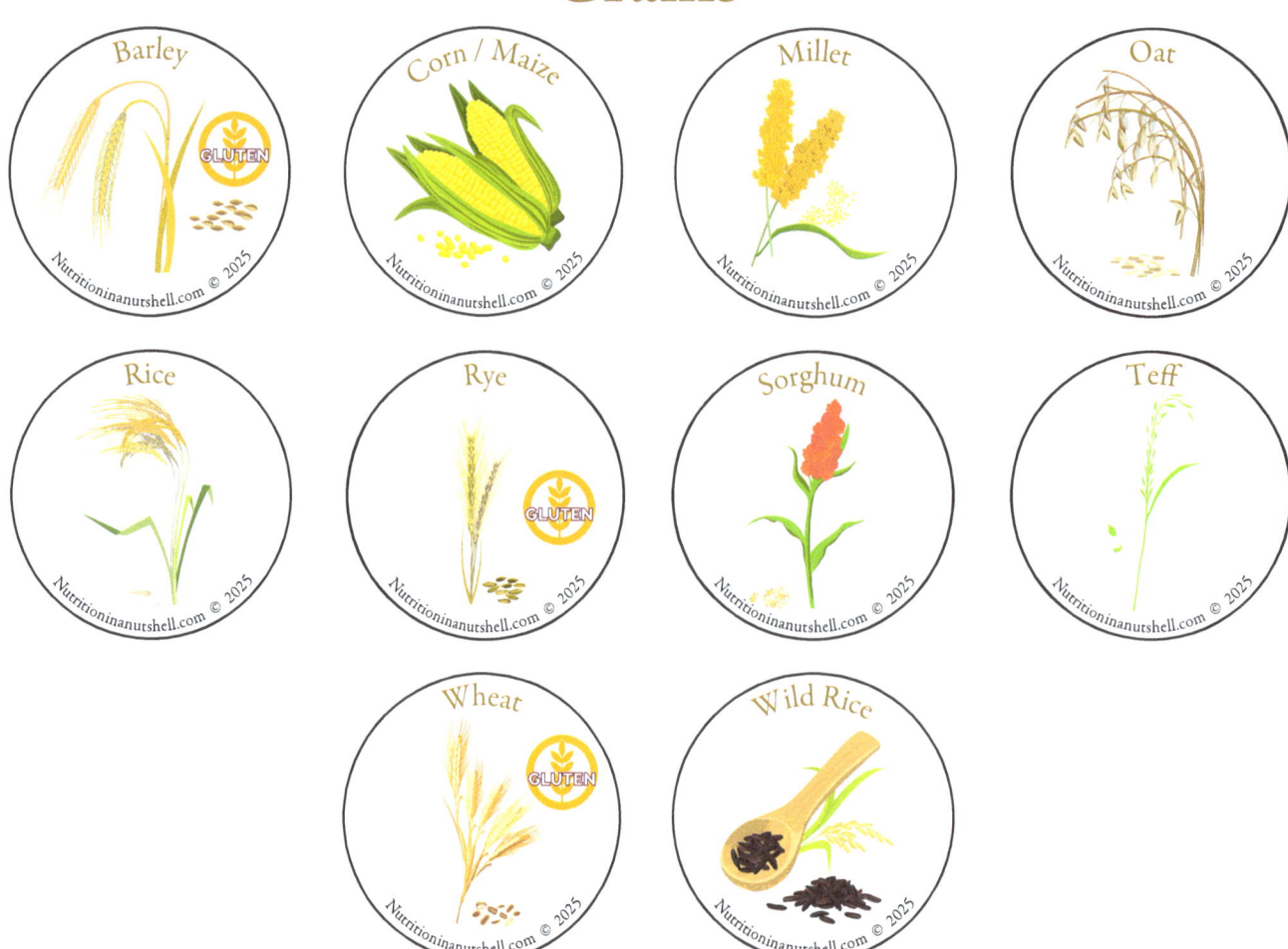

Legumes

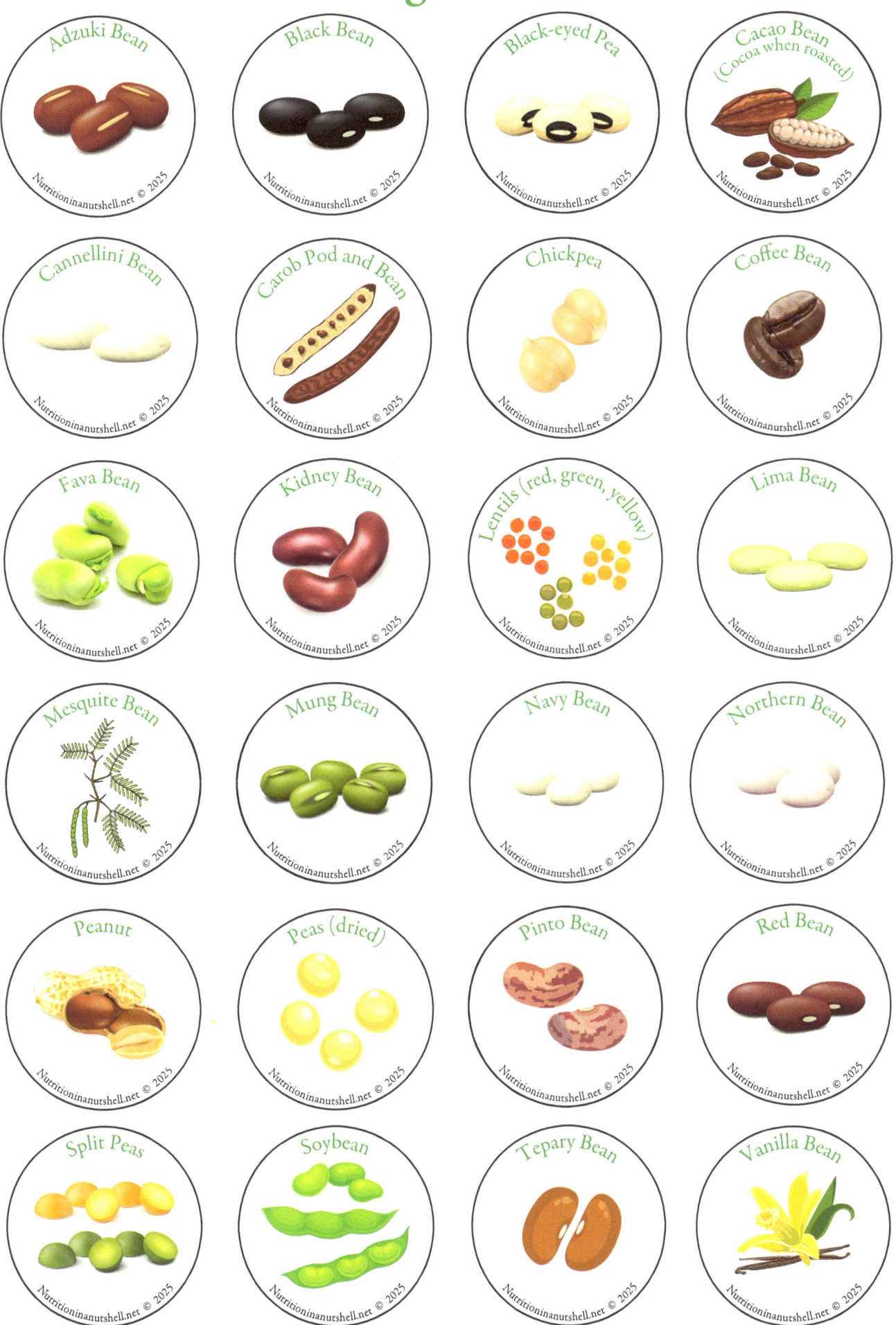

Tree Nuts

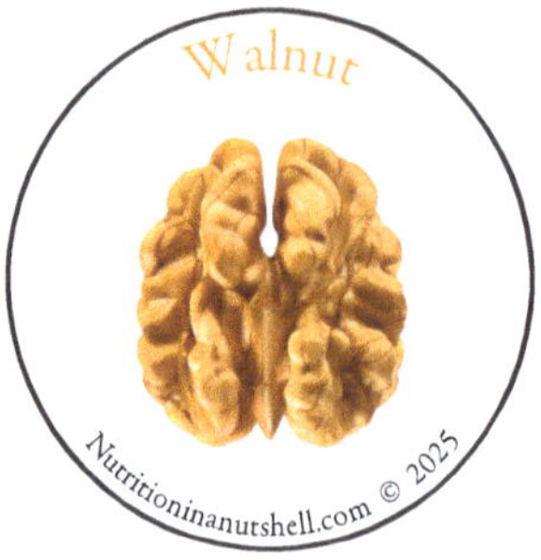

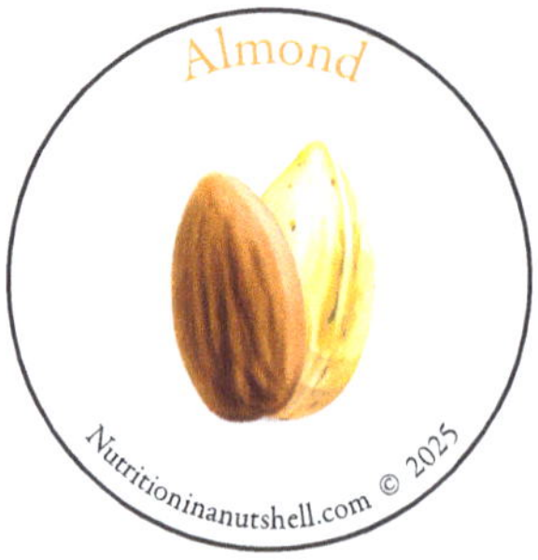

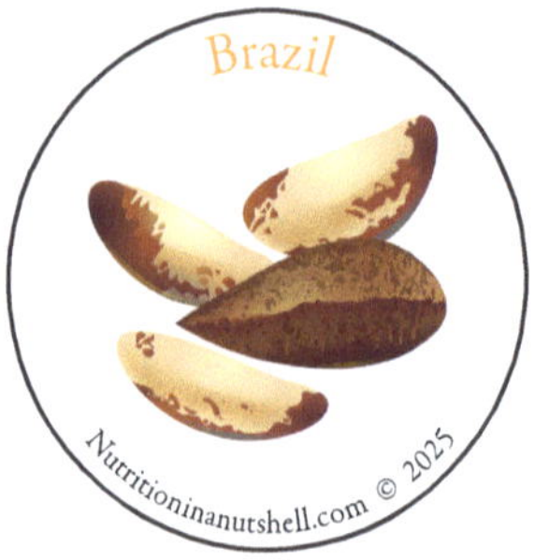

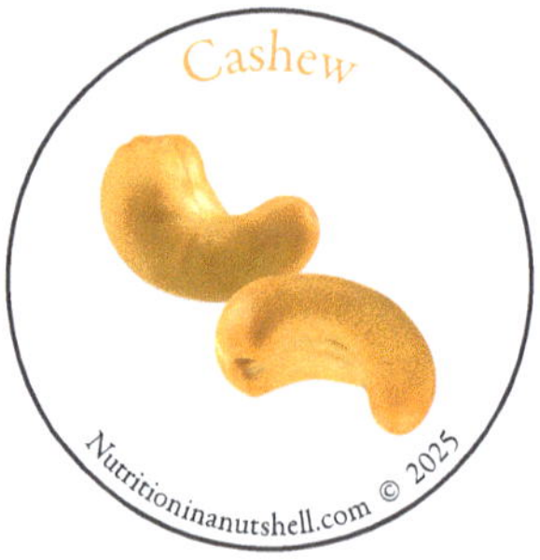

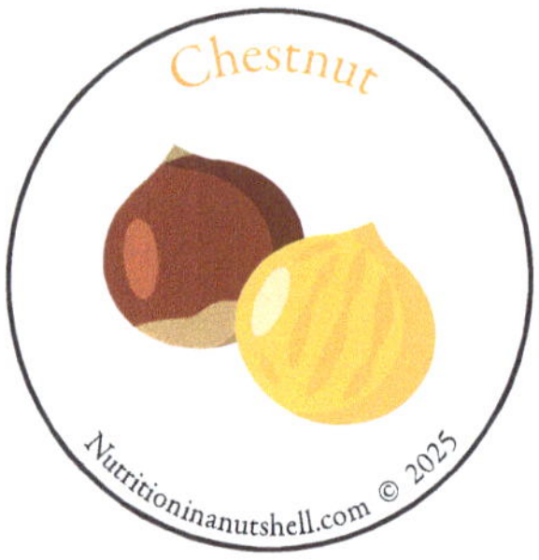

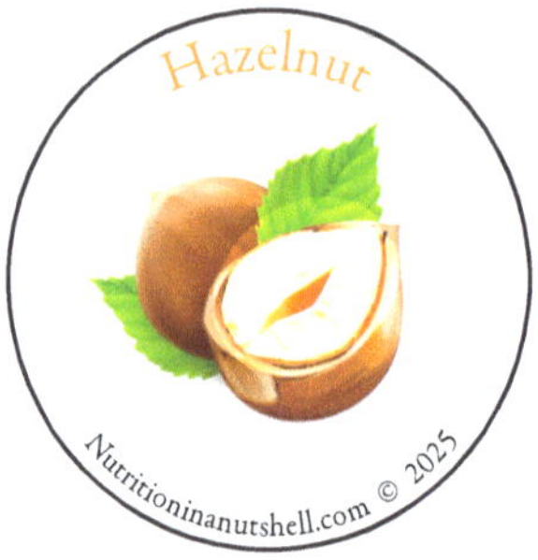

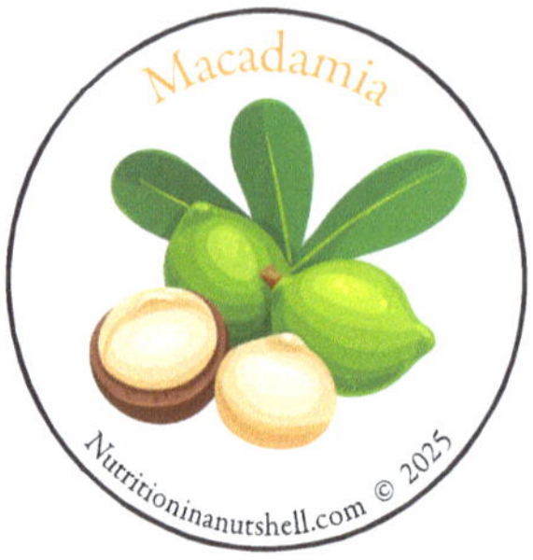

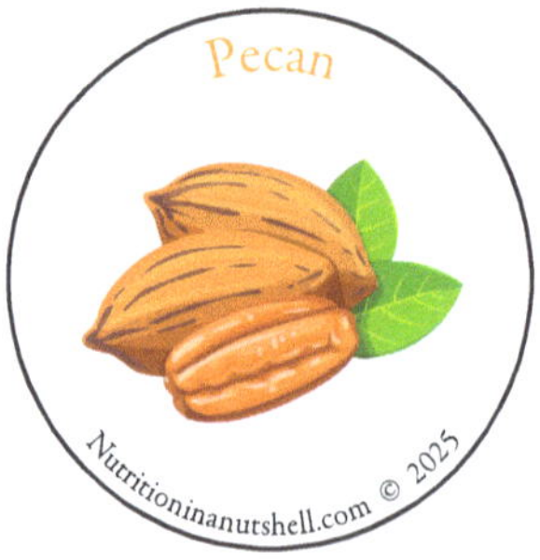

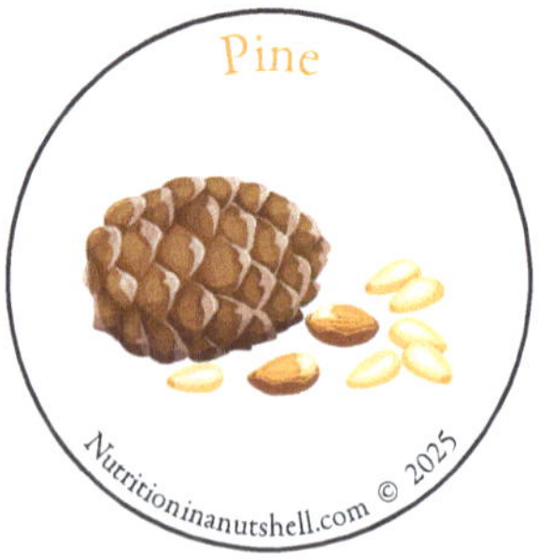

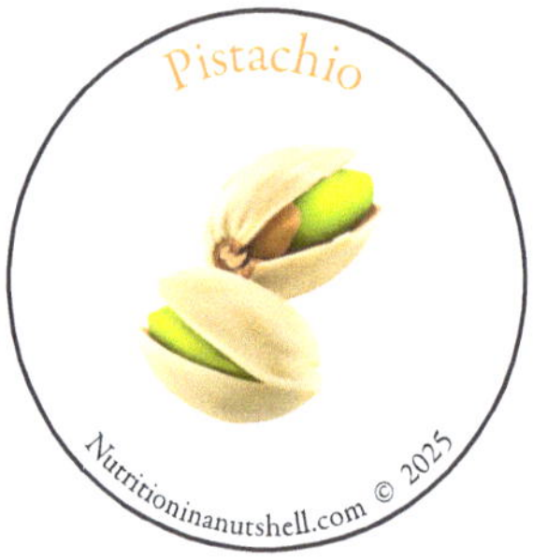

- Almond
- Brazil
- Cashew
- Chestnut
- Hazelnut
- Macadamia
- Pecan
- Pine
- Pistachio
- Walnut

Bark & Saps

- Cinnamon Bark
- Beech Tree Syrup
- Birch Tree Syrup
- Hickory Tree Syrup
- Maple Syrup
- Walnut Tree Syrup

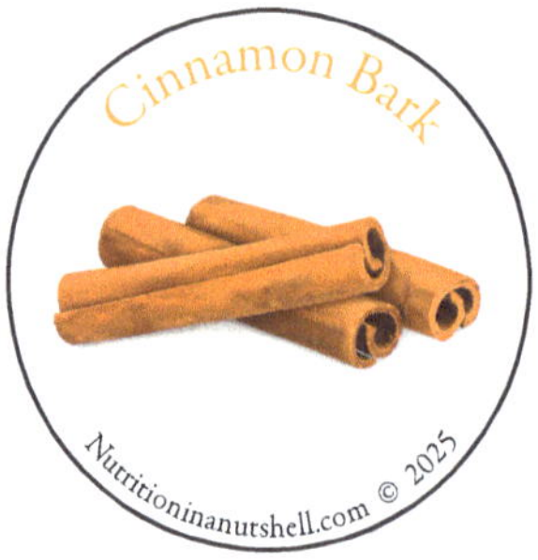

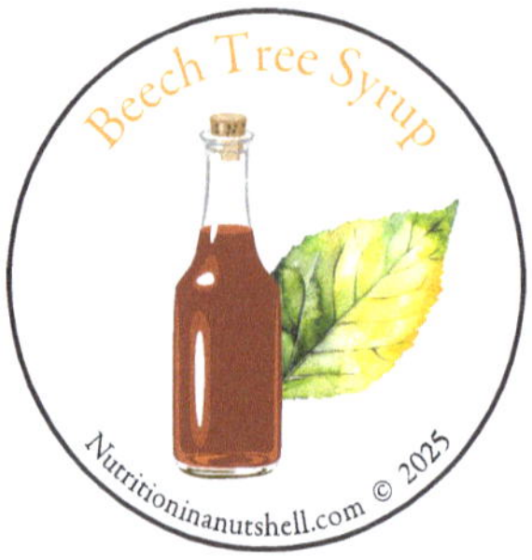

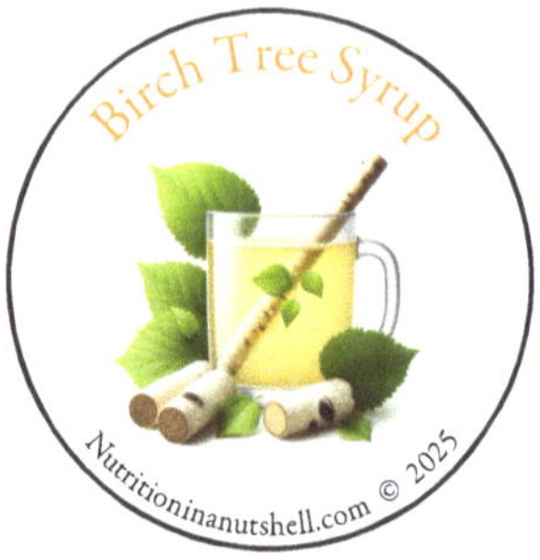

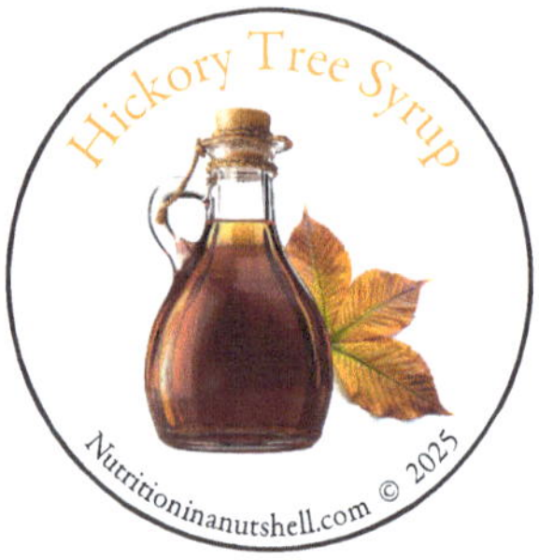

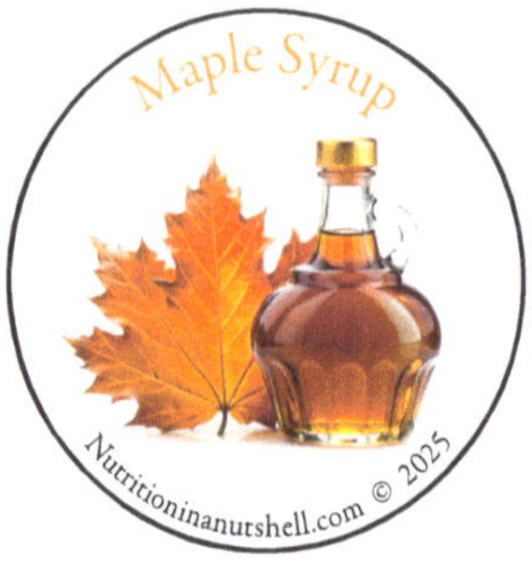

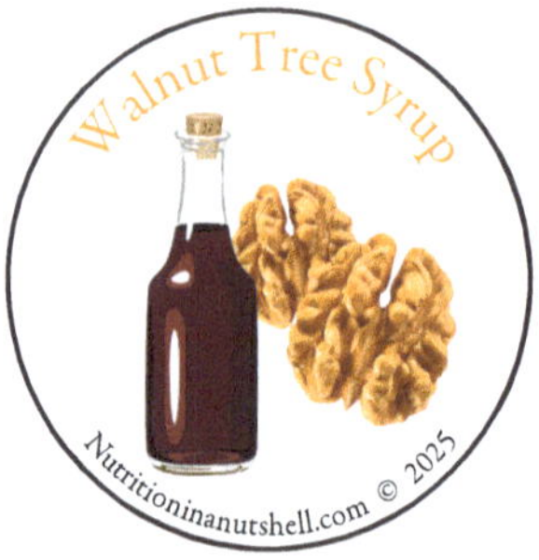

Seeds

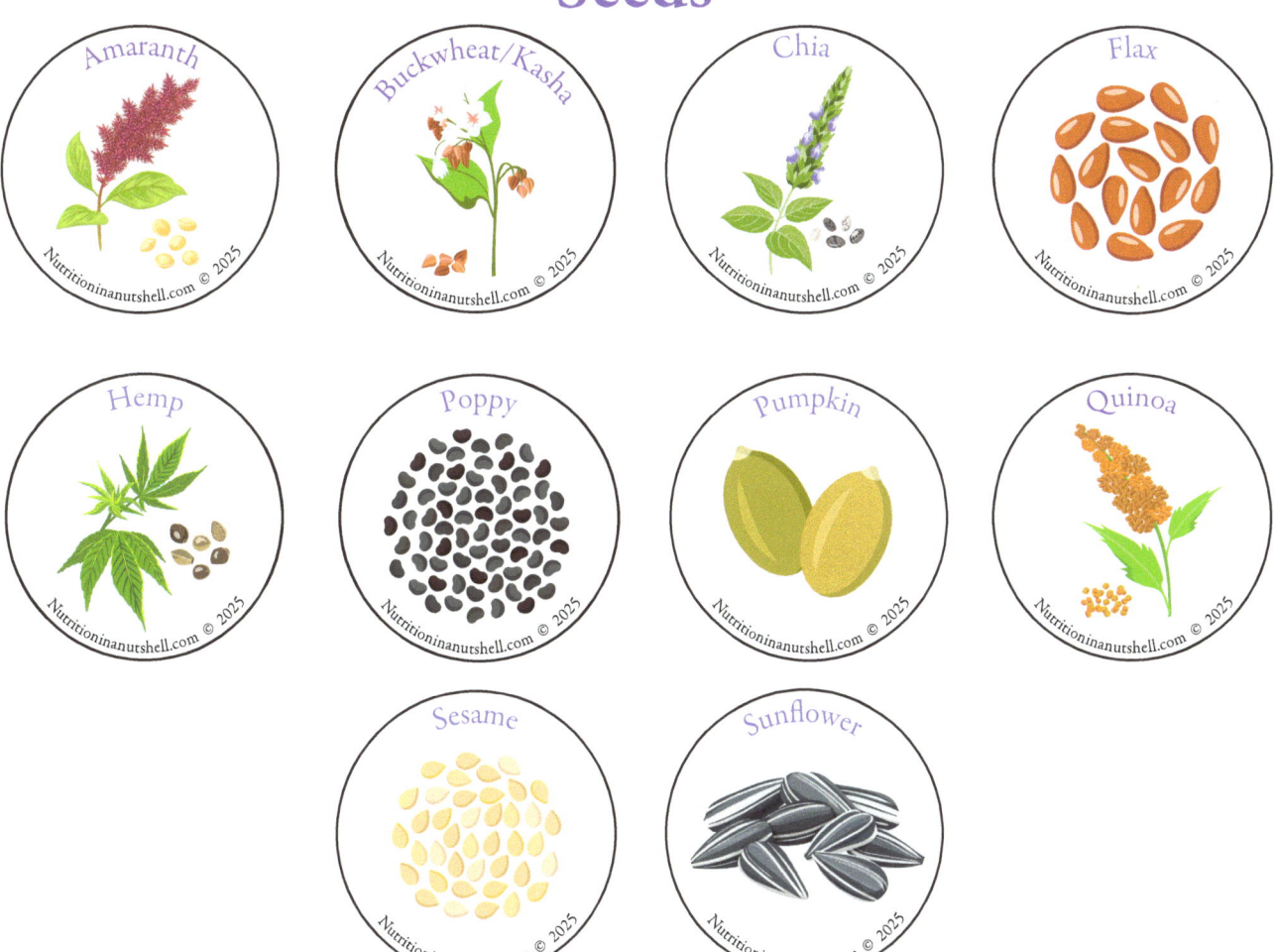

Seasonings

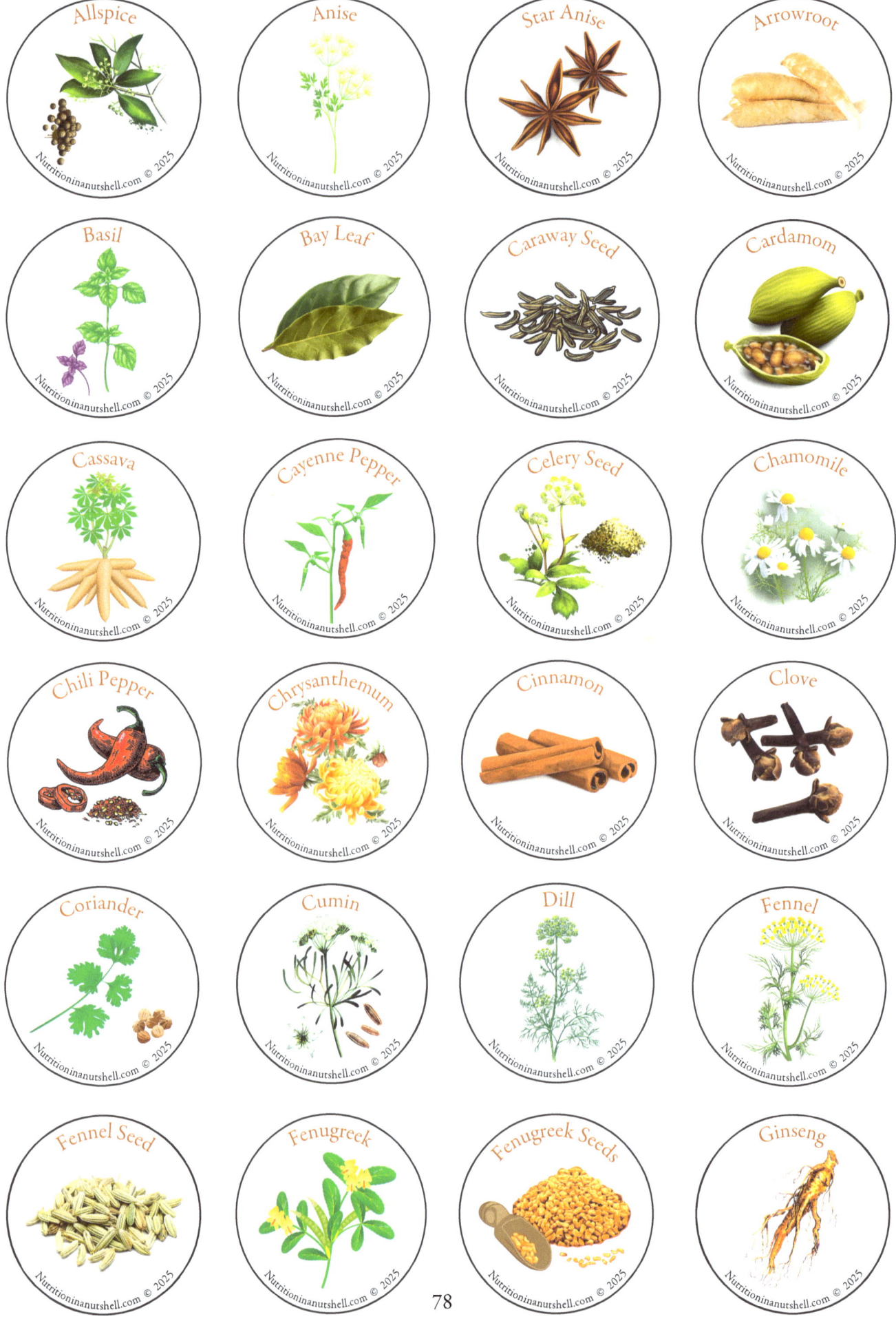

Seasonings

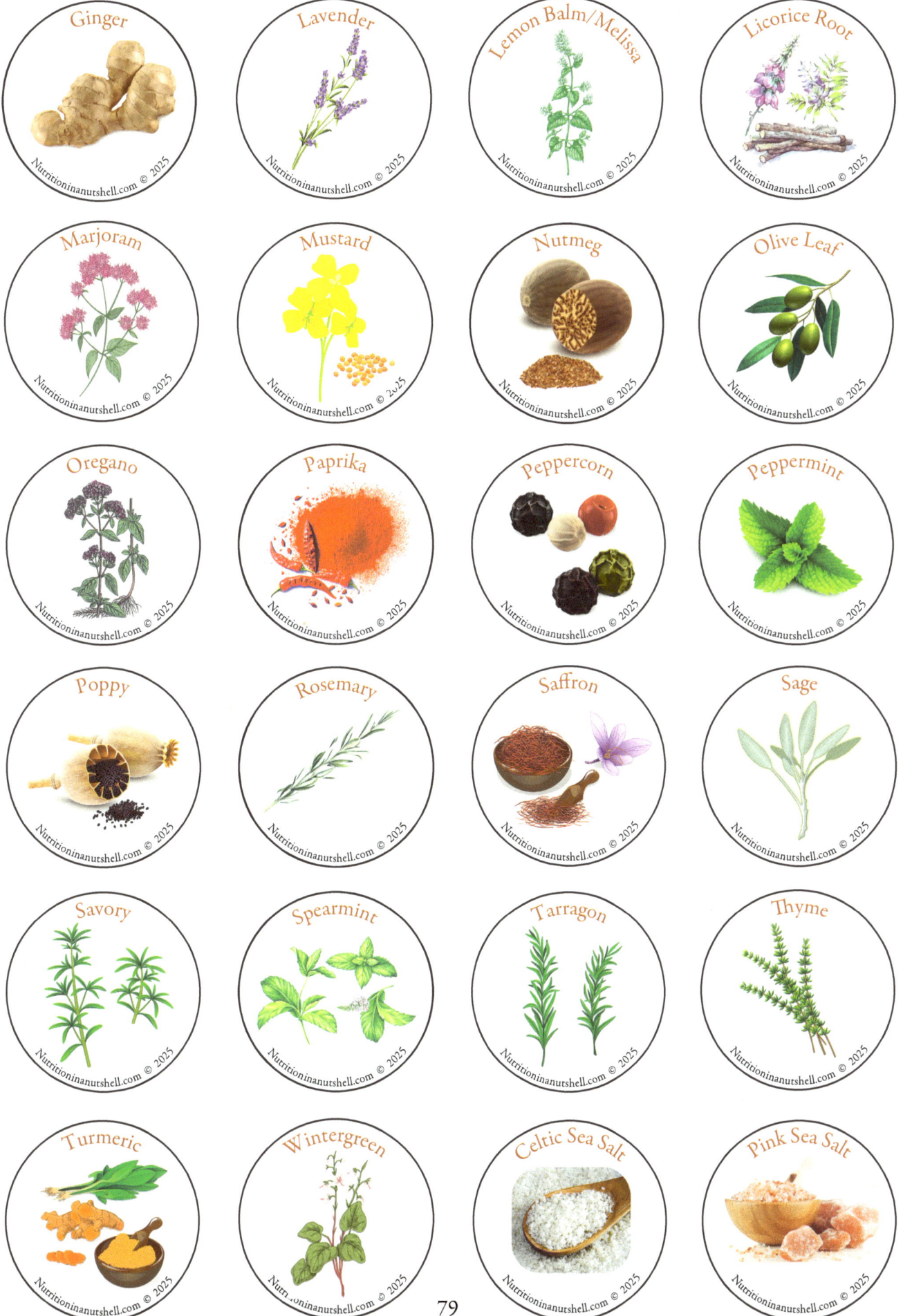

Vegetables

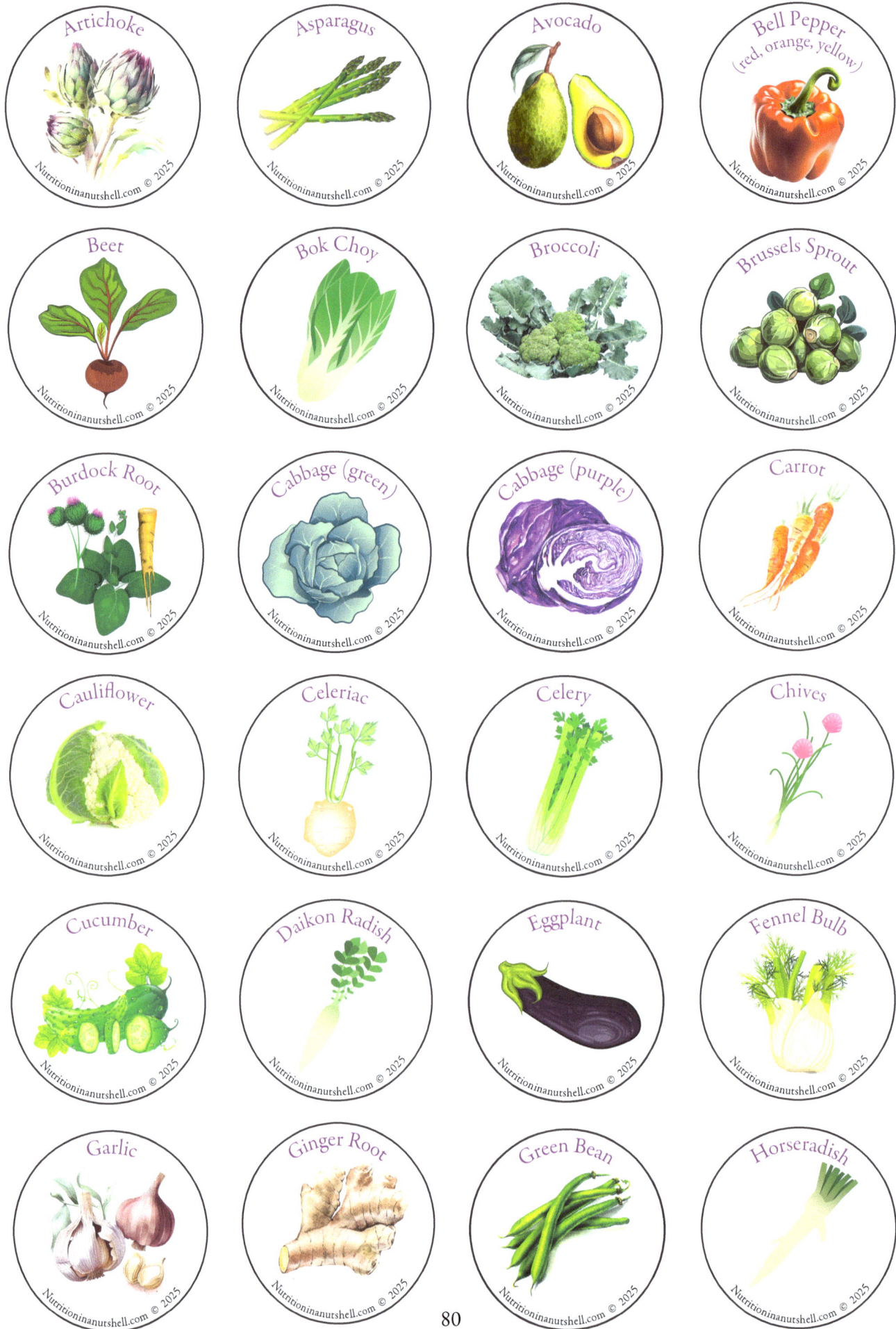

Vegetables

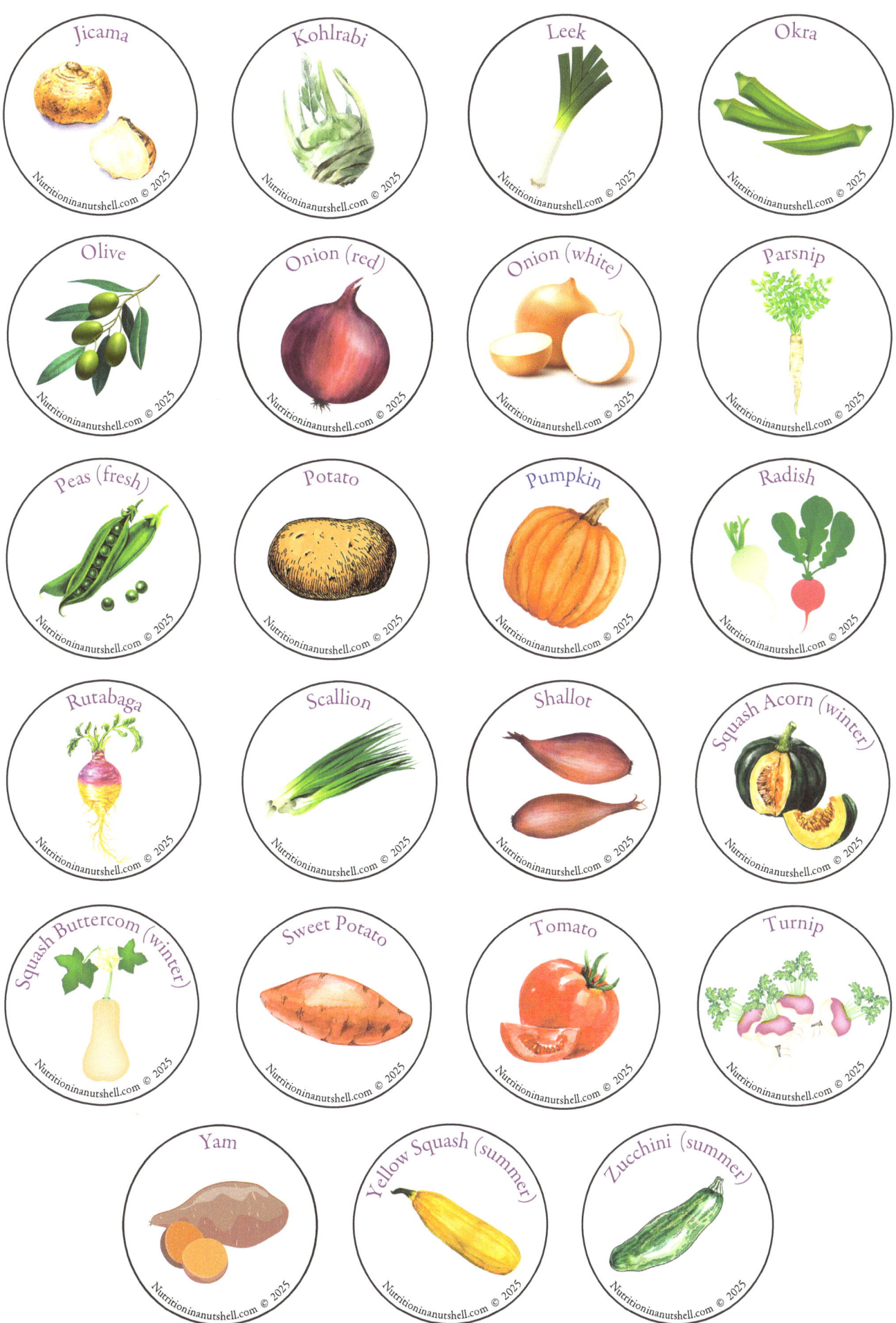

Leafy Greens

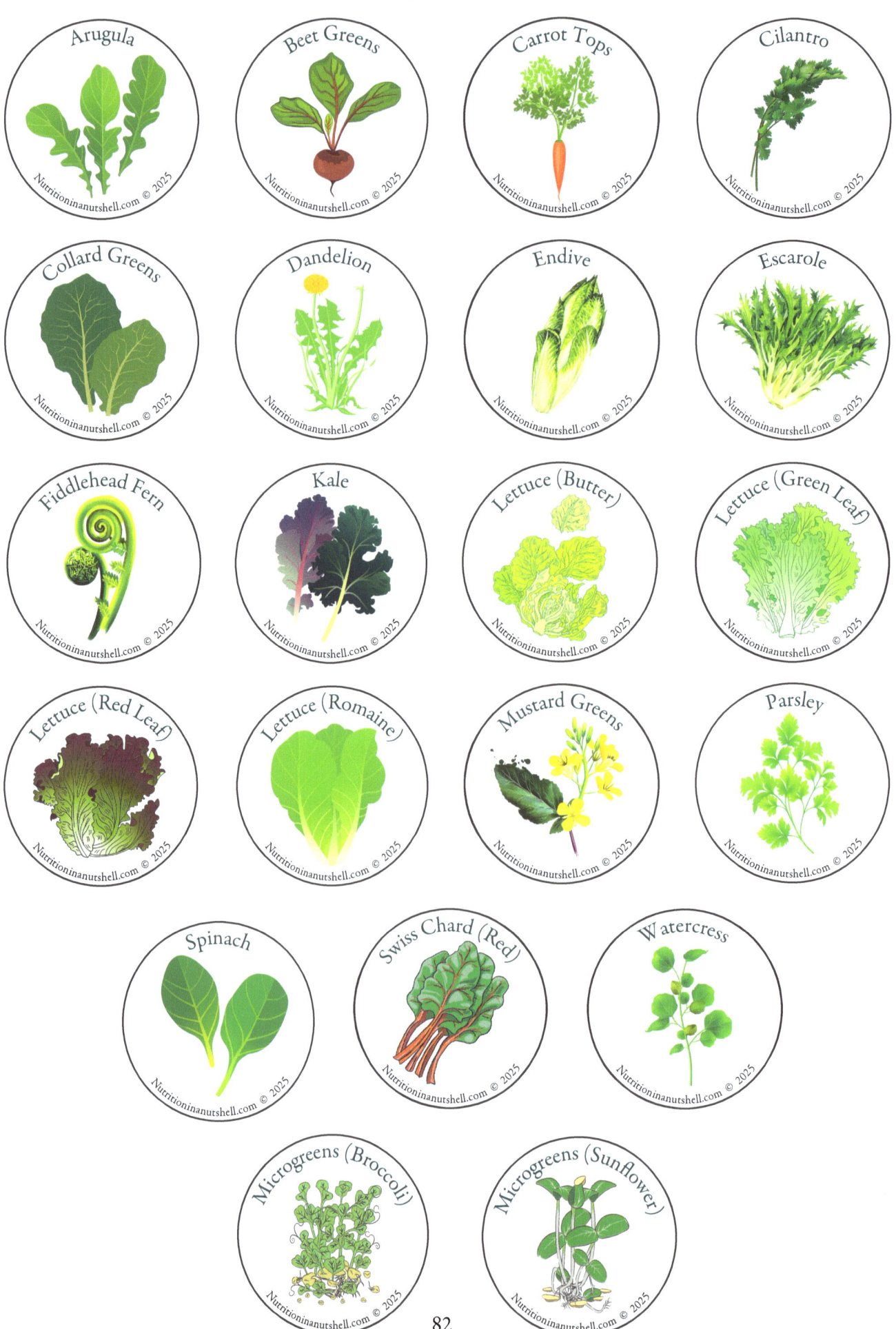

Plant Oils

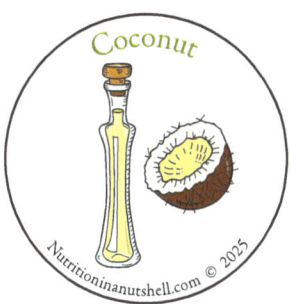
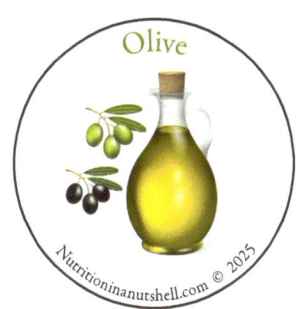

Mushrooms

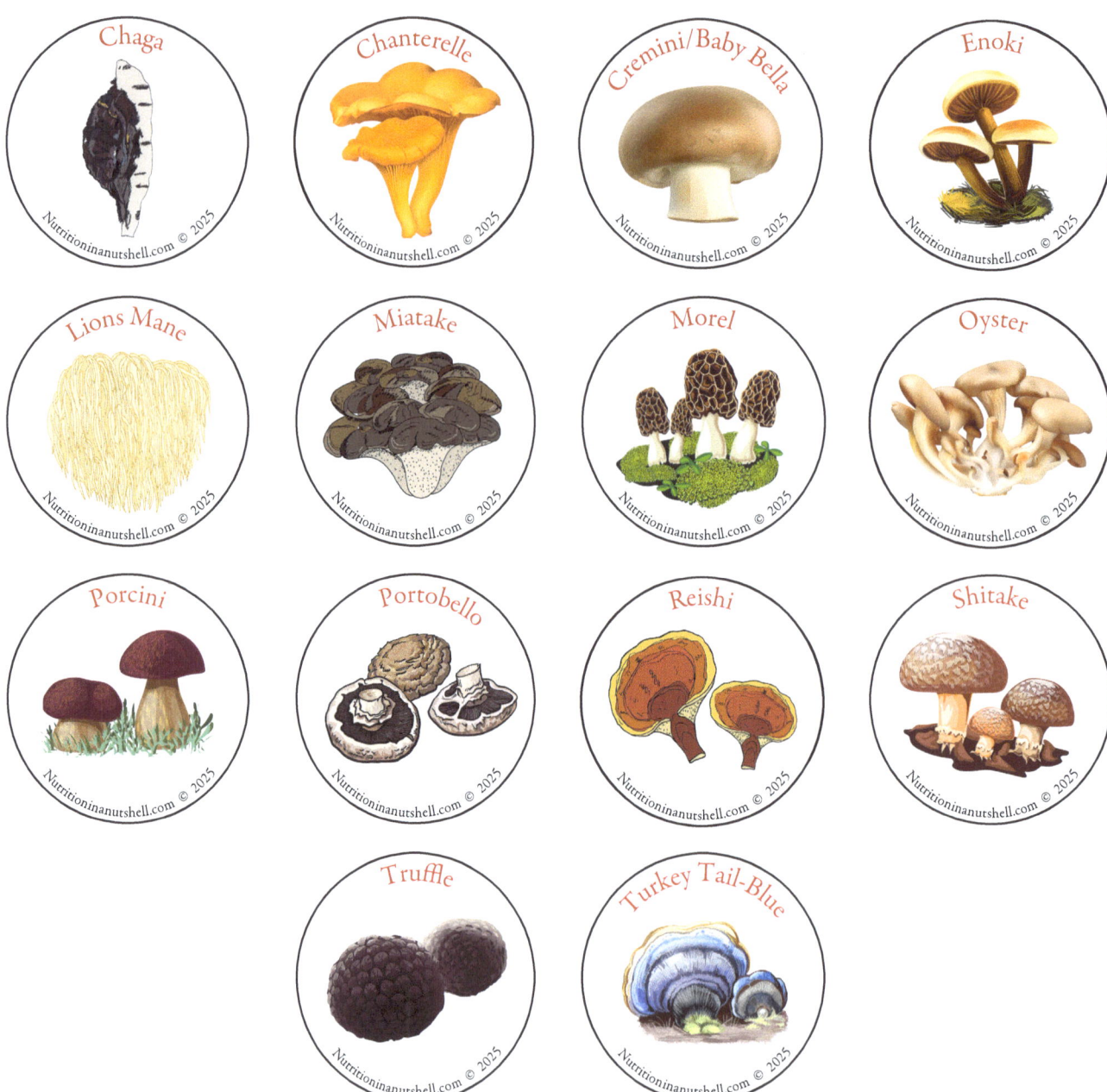

Seaweeds & Chlorella (Algae)

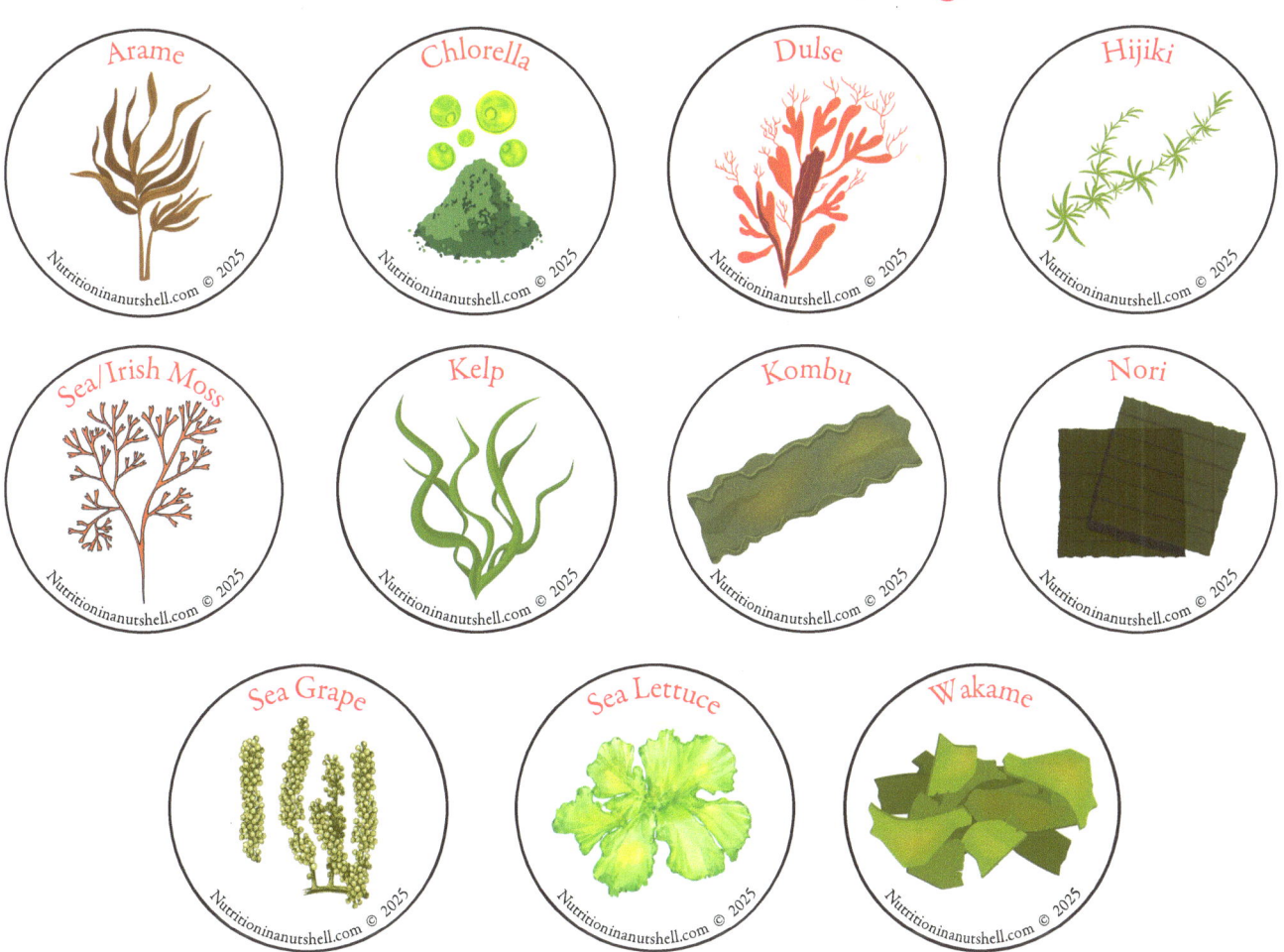

Cyanobacteria

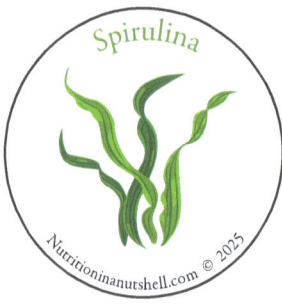 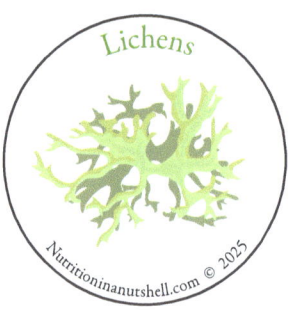

Spirulina is an ancient photosynthesizing single-celled bacteria that lives in colonies, inhabiting fresh and saltwater ecosystems. Although spirulina is part of the *Bacteria* Kingdom, it has similar attributes to algae and is, therefore, often thought of as blue-green algae.

Lichen is generally used for medicinal purposes rather than as a food because it can cause indigestion; and lichen should only be harvested from pristine environments because it easily absorbs pollutants.

Probiotic Ferments (Bacteria & Fungi)

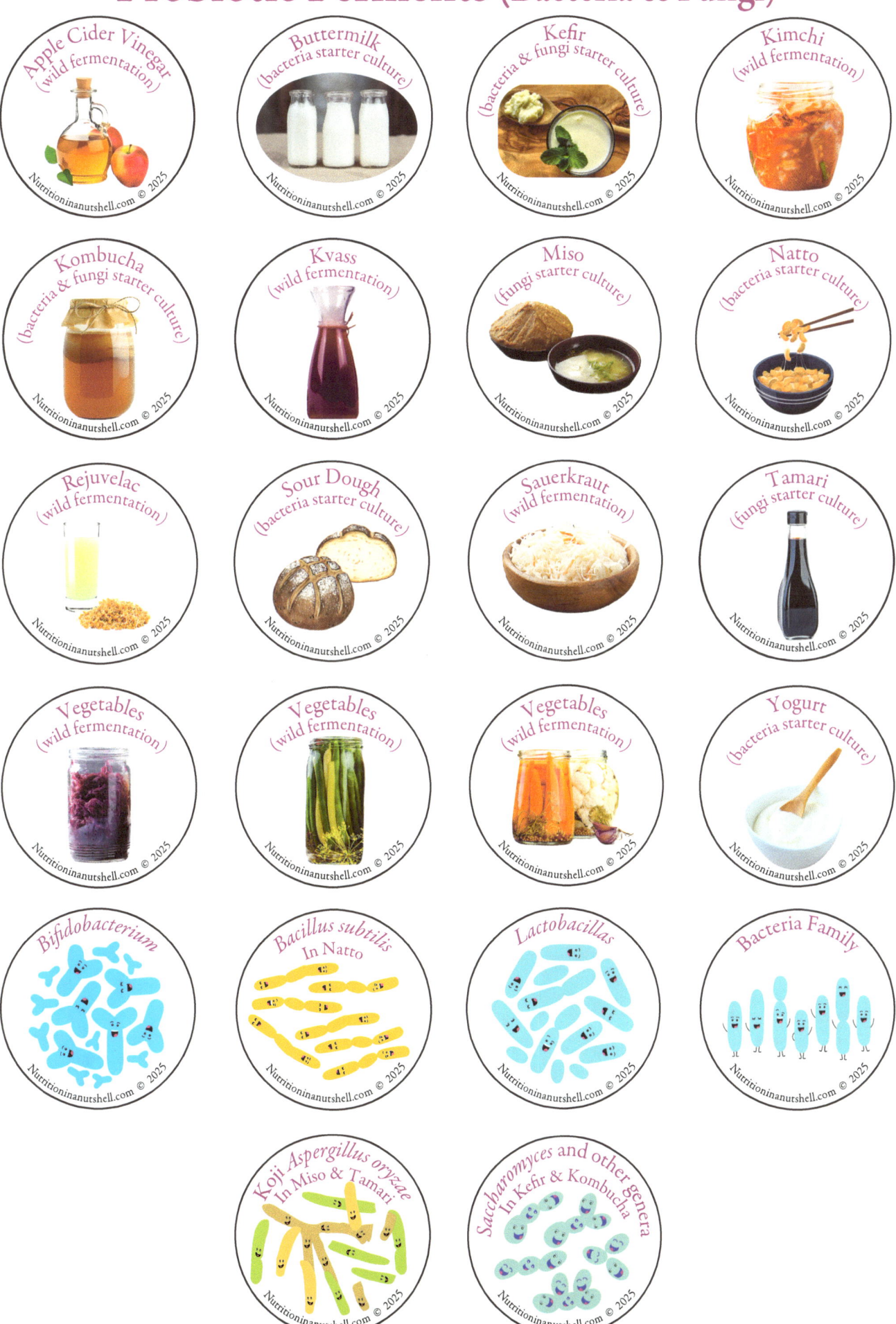

Preparing Natural Foods Traditionally

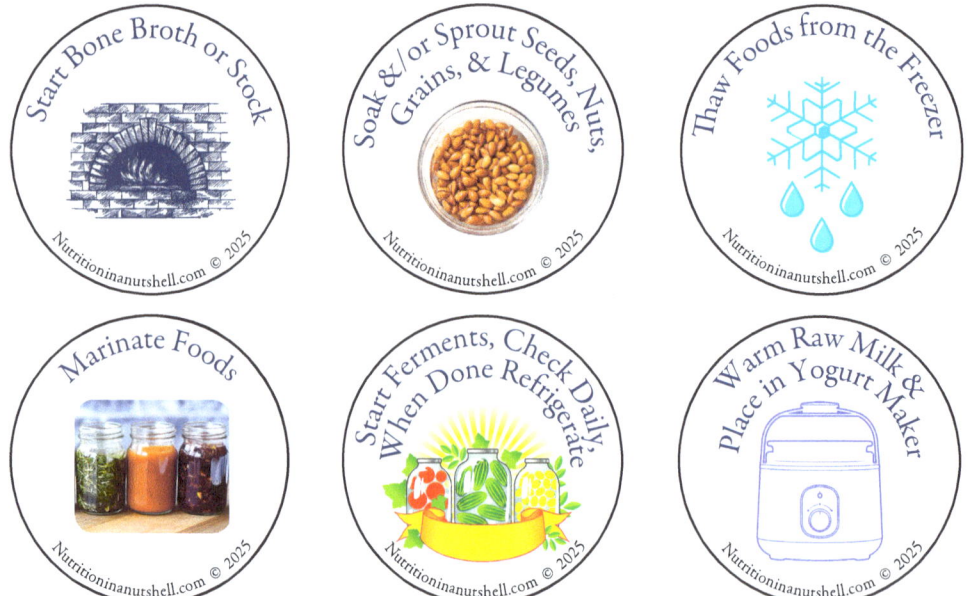

Natural Living

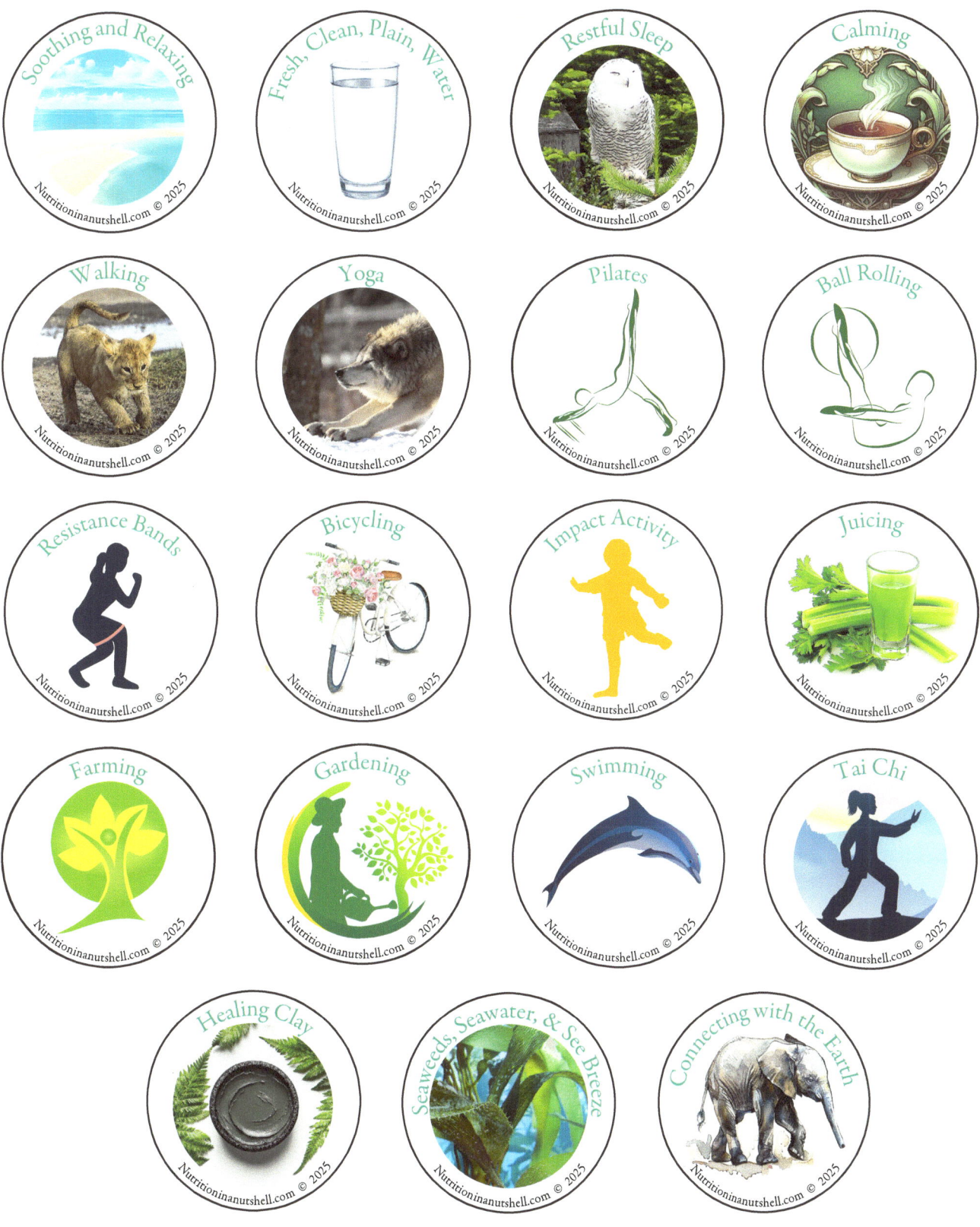

With great appreciation to the Artists who contributed to these ACTIVITY BOOK materials – photos and illustrations

From ©Shutterstock.com
Wooden Plate by Dea Indah Purnama

From ©Dreamstime.com
Wooden Bowl by Gl0ck33
Wooden Cutting Board by Patarajan
Stock Pot by Alexander Babich
Blender and Juicers by Kamenuka
Clay Pot by Bert Folsom
Window Box and Raised Bed by Kinek00

Natural Foods
from the Tapestry *of* Life
ACTIVITY BOOK
Materials

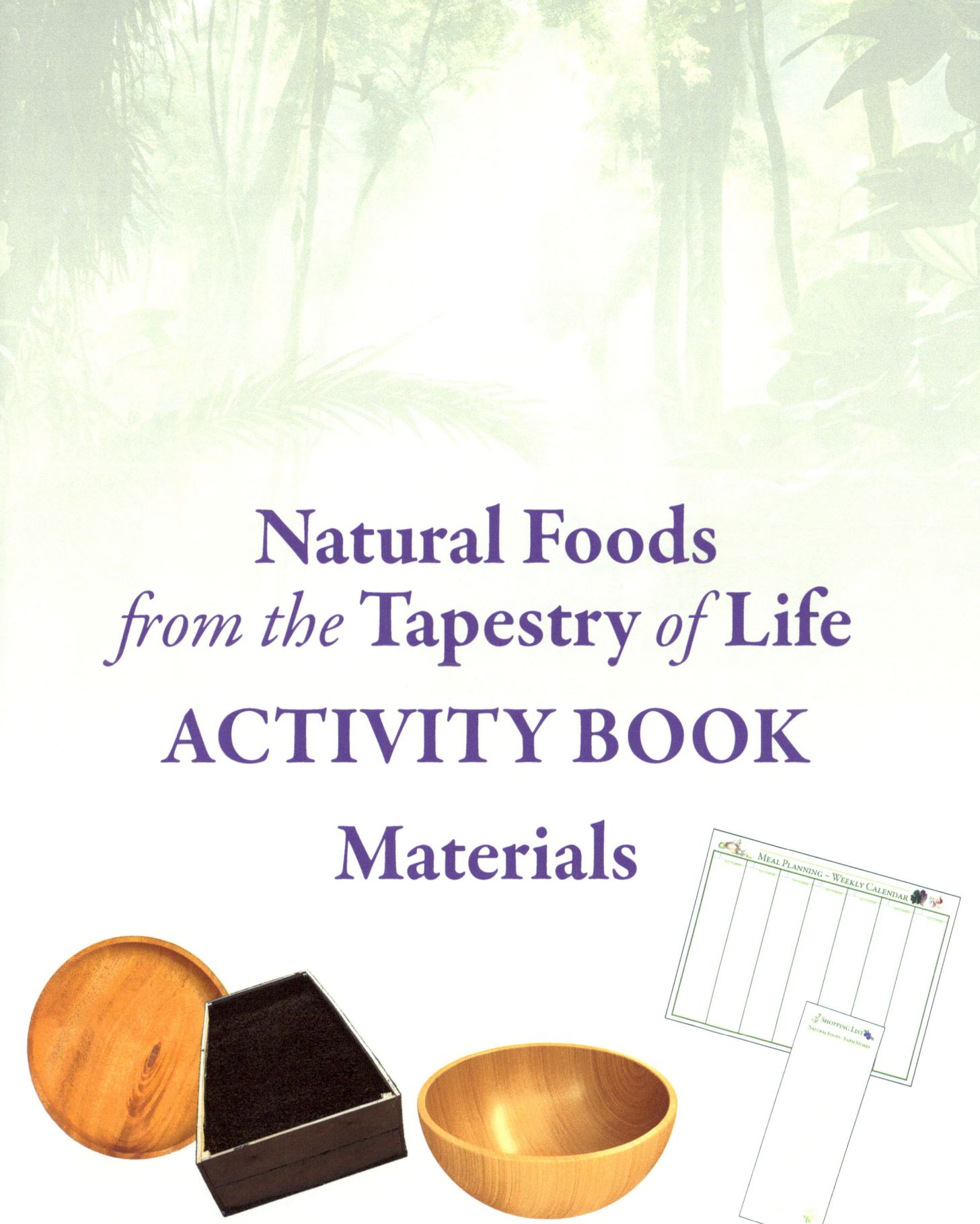

3 Practical Steps, Educational Activities #19 & 21

Meal Planning – Weekly Calendar

| DAY OF WEEK |
| DAY OF WEEK |
| DAY OF WEEK |
| DAY OF WEEK |
| DAY OF WEEK |
| DAY OF WEEK |
| DAY OF WEEK |

SHOPPING LIST

Natural Foods | Farm Stores

SHOPPING LIST

Natural Foods | Farm Stores

3 Practical Steps

Educational Activity #18

PLATE for Meal Planning

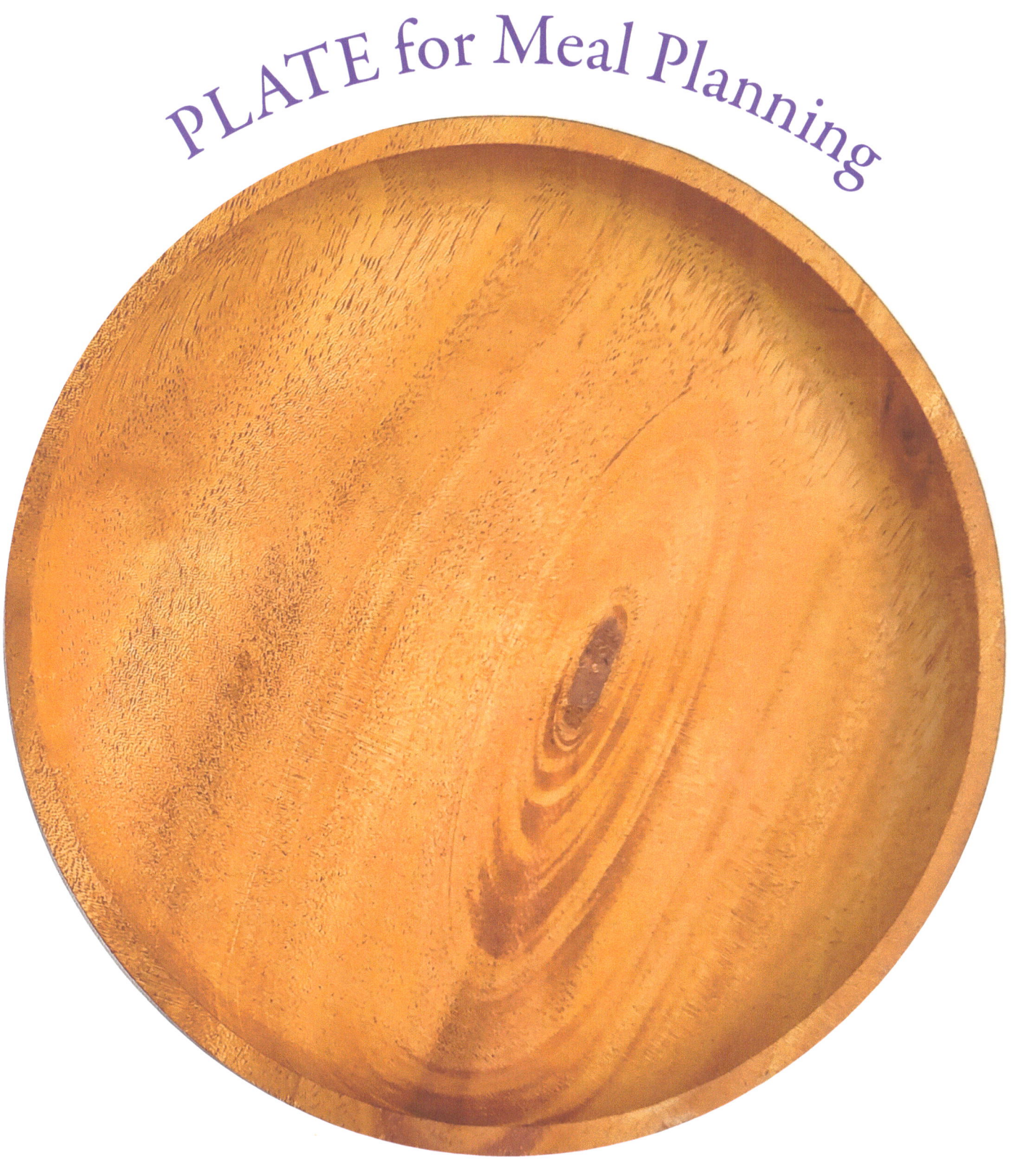

Educational Activity #18

SMALL BOWL for Meal Planning

Educational Activity #18

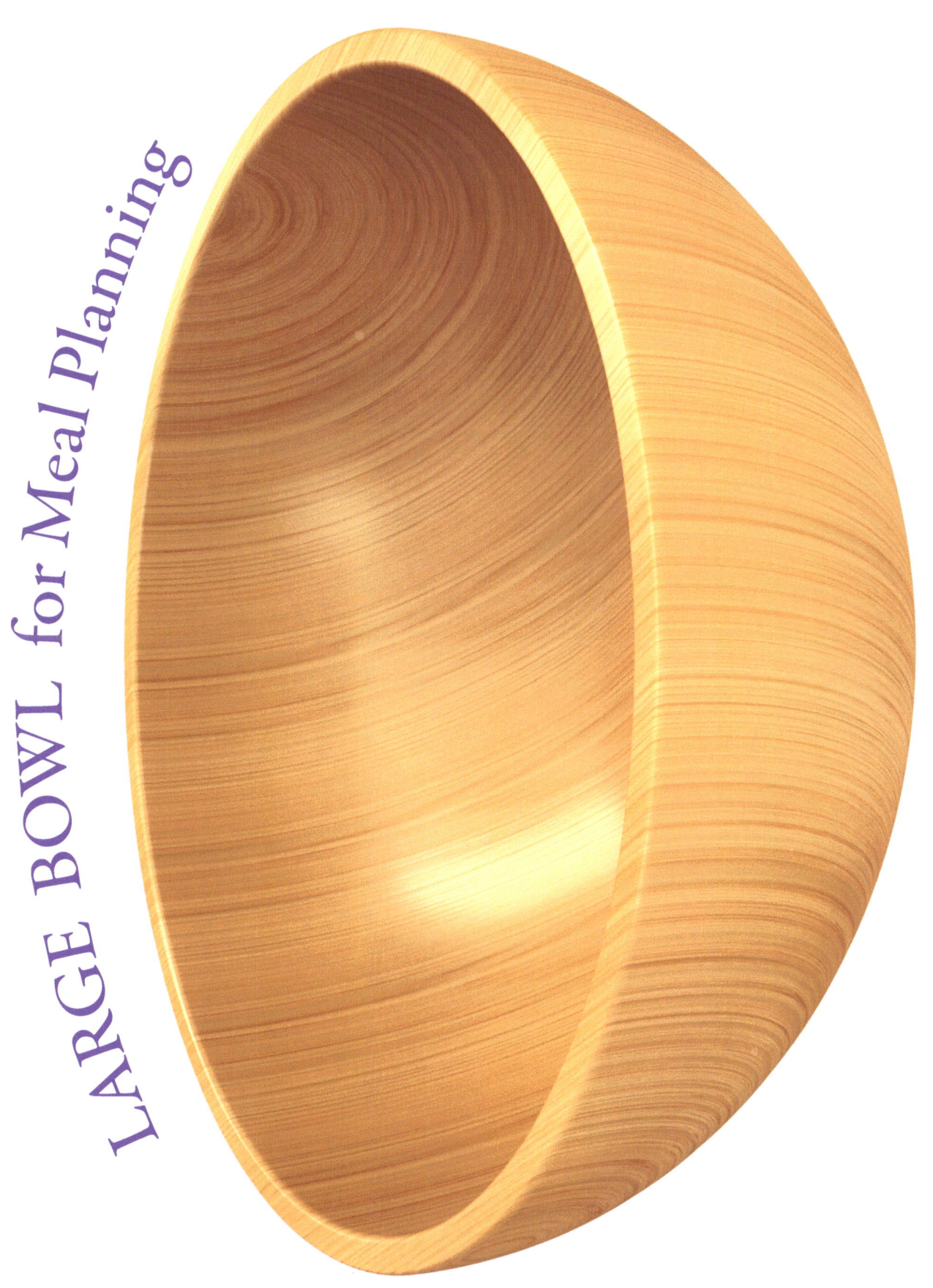

LARGE BOWL for Meal Planning

Educational Activity #18

CHARCUTERIE BOARD for Meal Planning

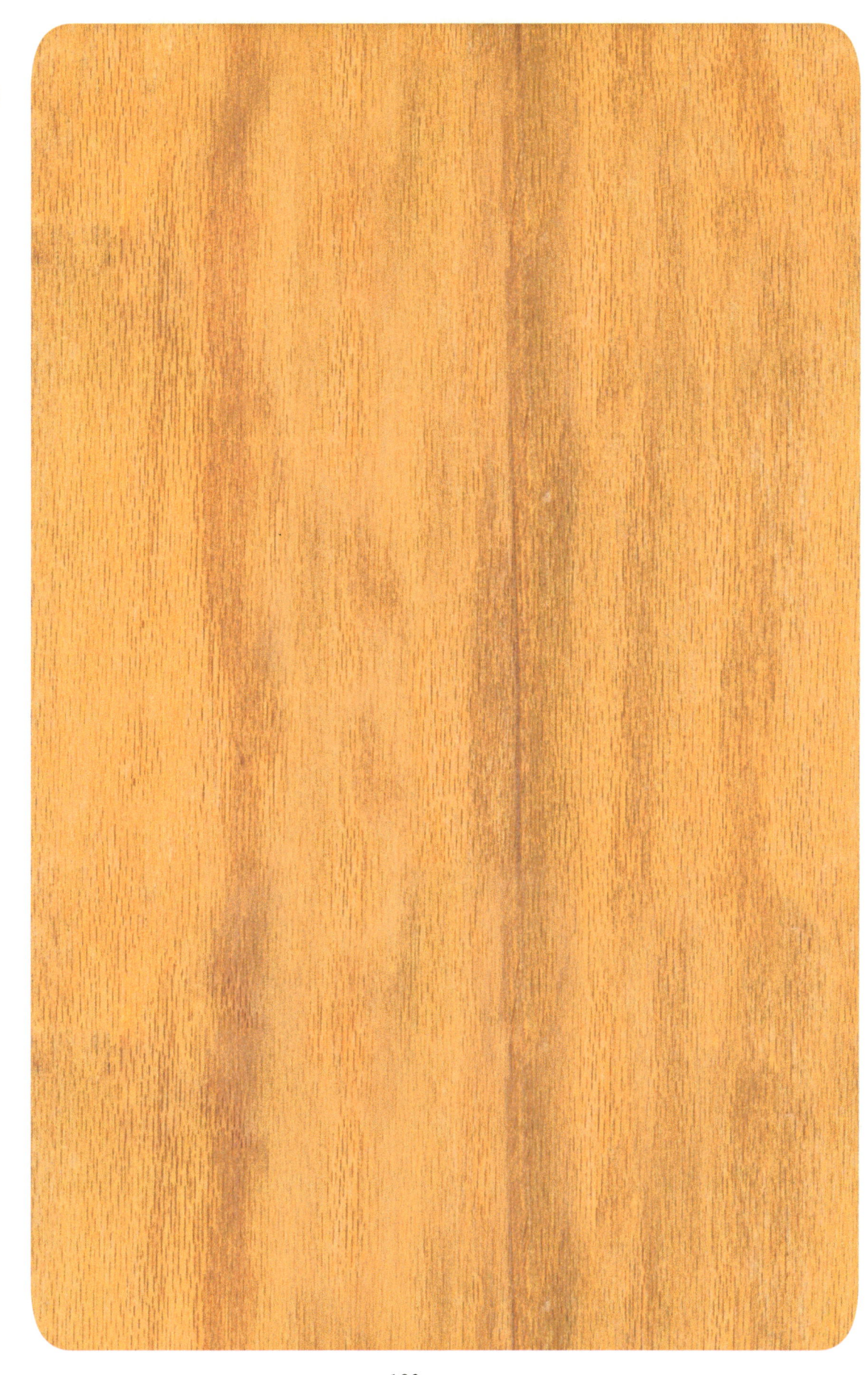

LARGE POT for Making Soup Stock and Bone Broth

Educational Activity #18

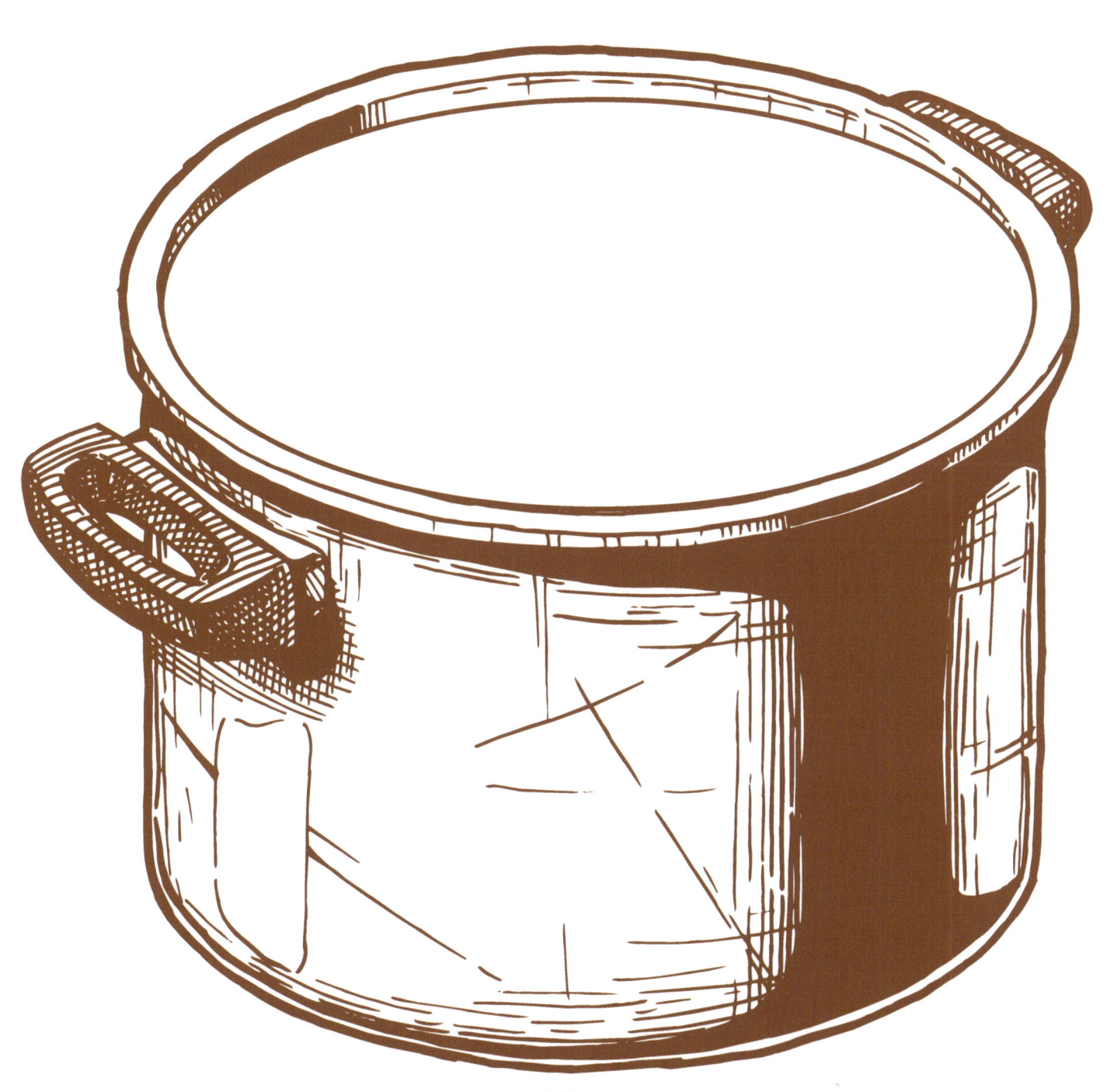

BLENDER for Meal Planning

Educational Activity #18

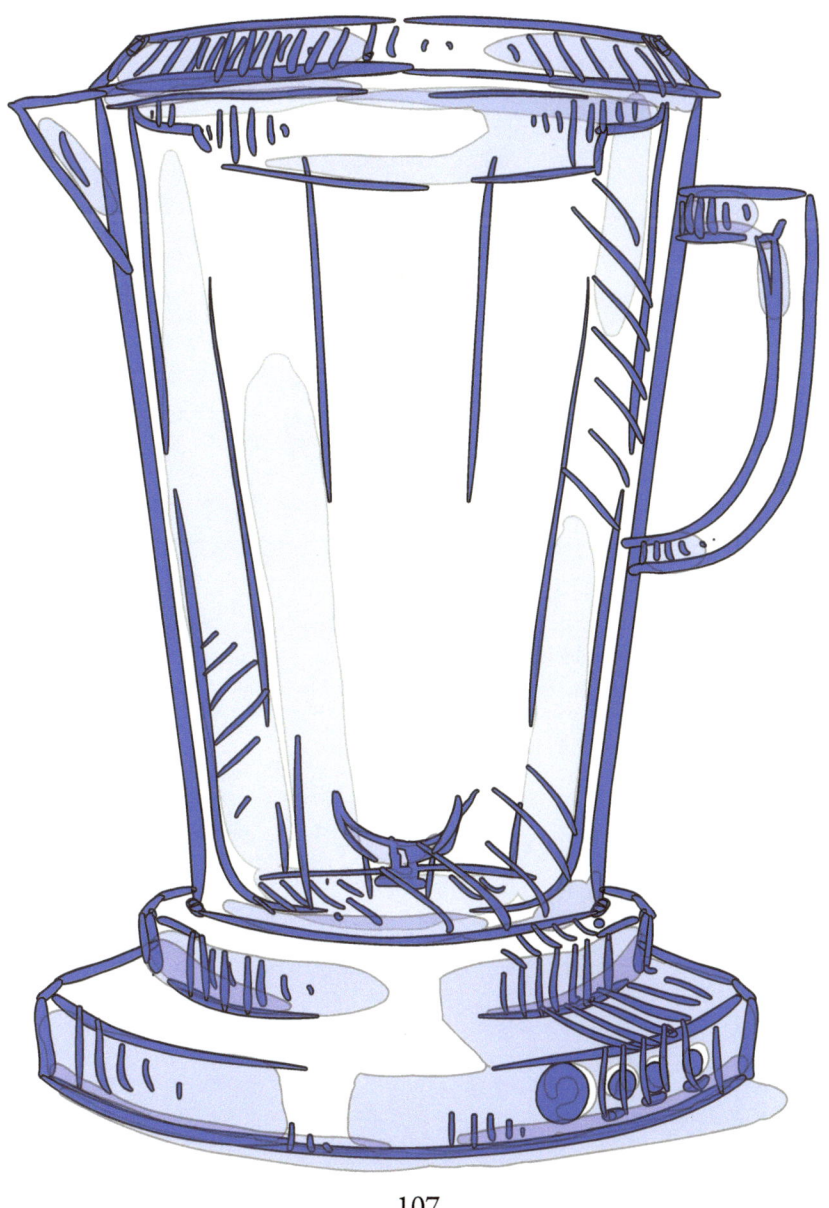

JUICER for Meal Planning

Educational Activity #18

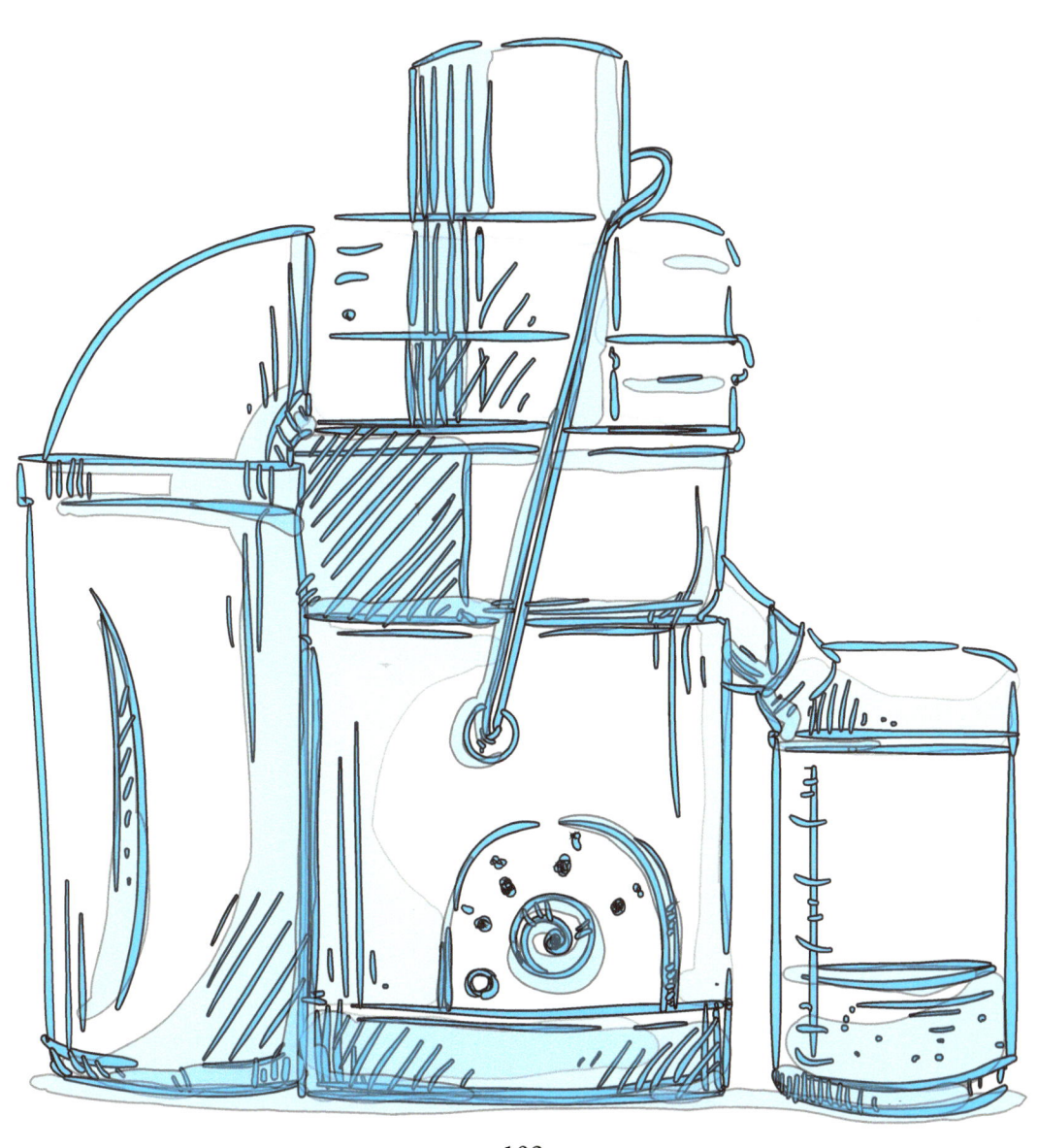

JUICER for Meal Planning

Educational Activity #18

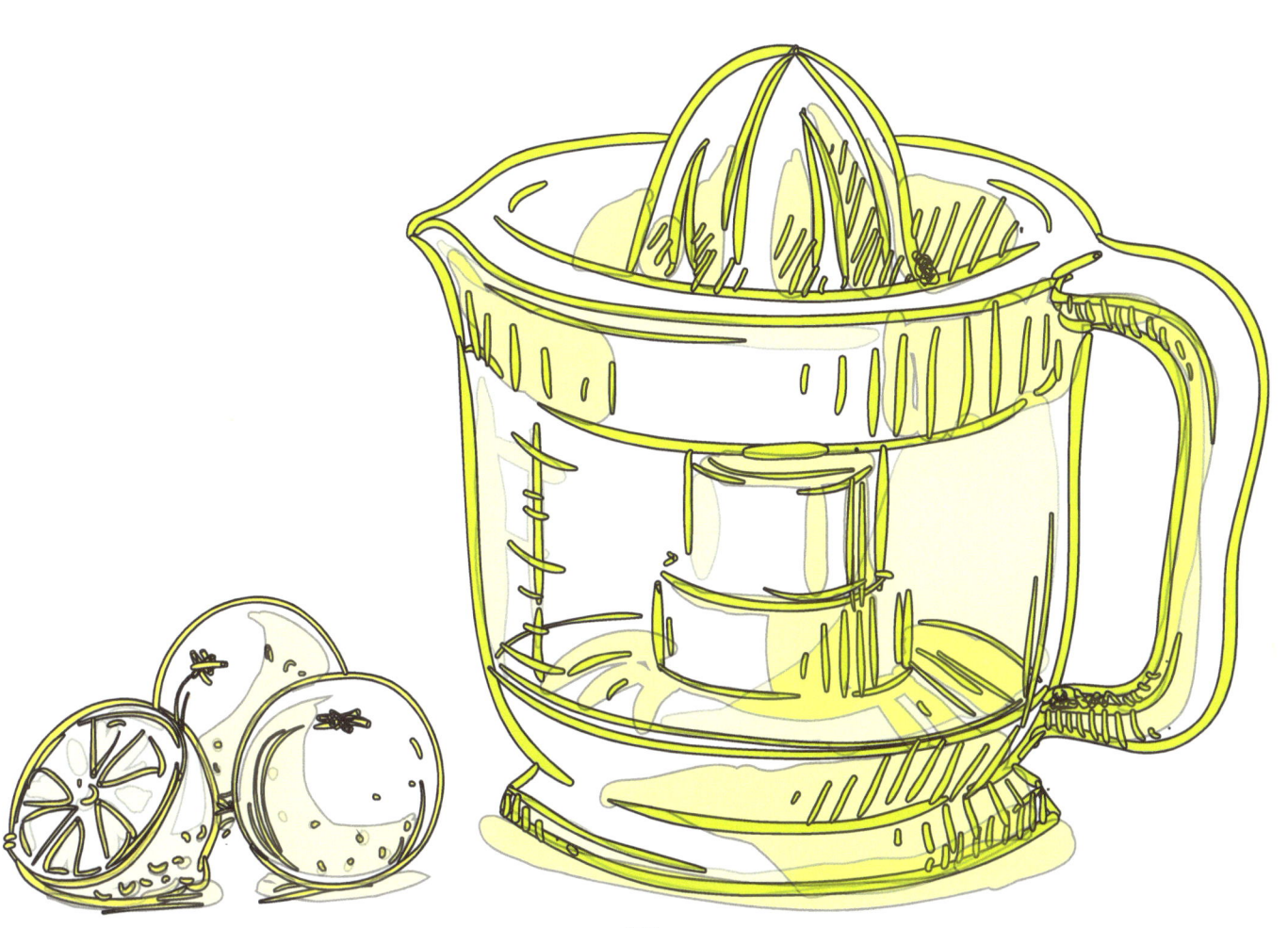

CLAY POT for Planting

Educational Activity #20

WINDOW BOX for Planting

Educational Activity #20

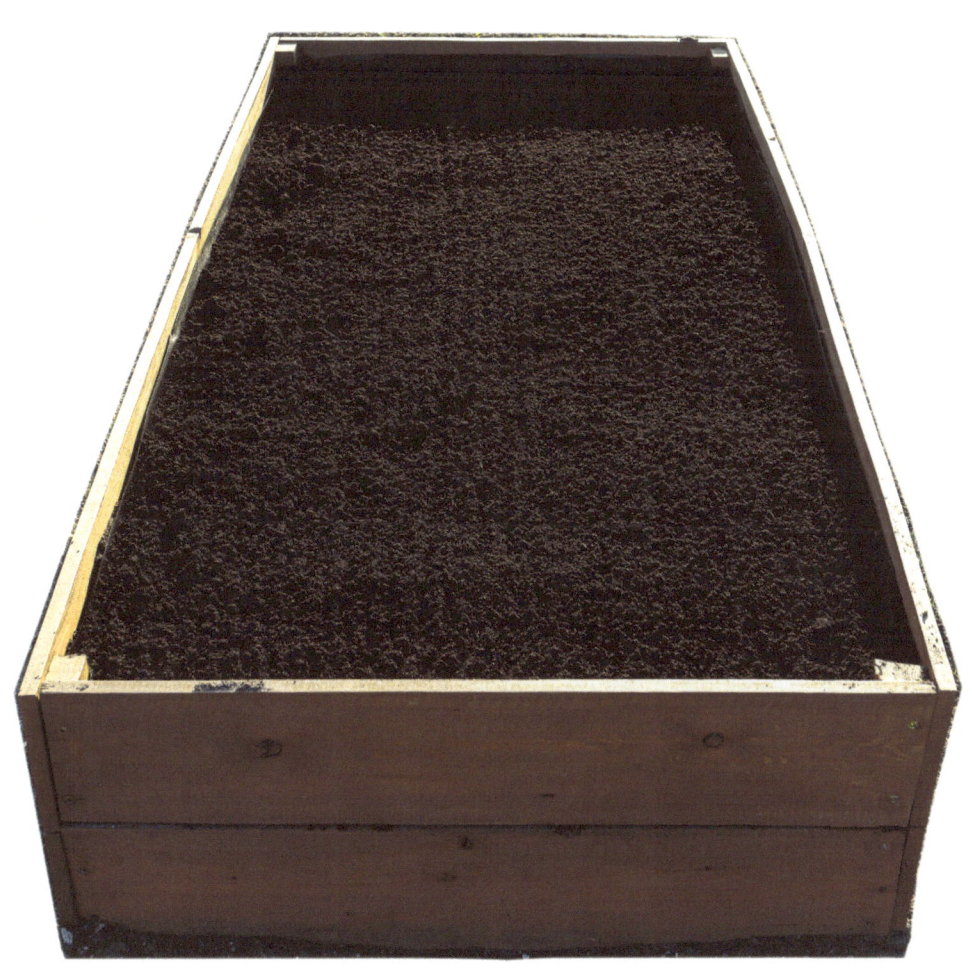

RAISED BED for Planting

Educational Activity #20

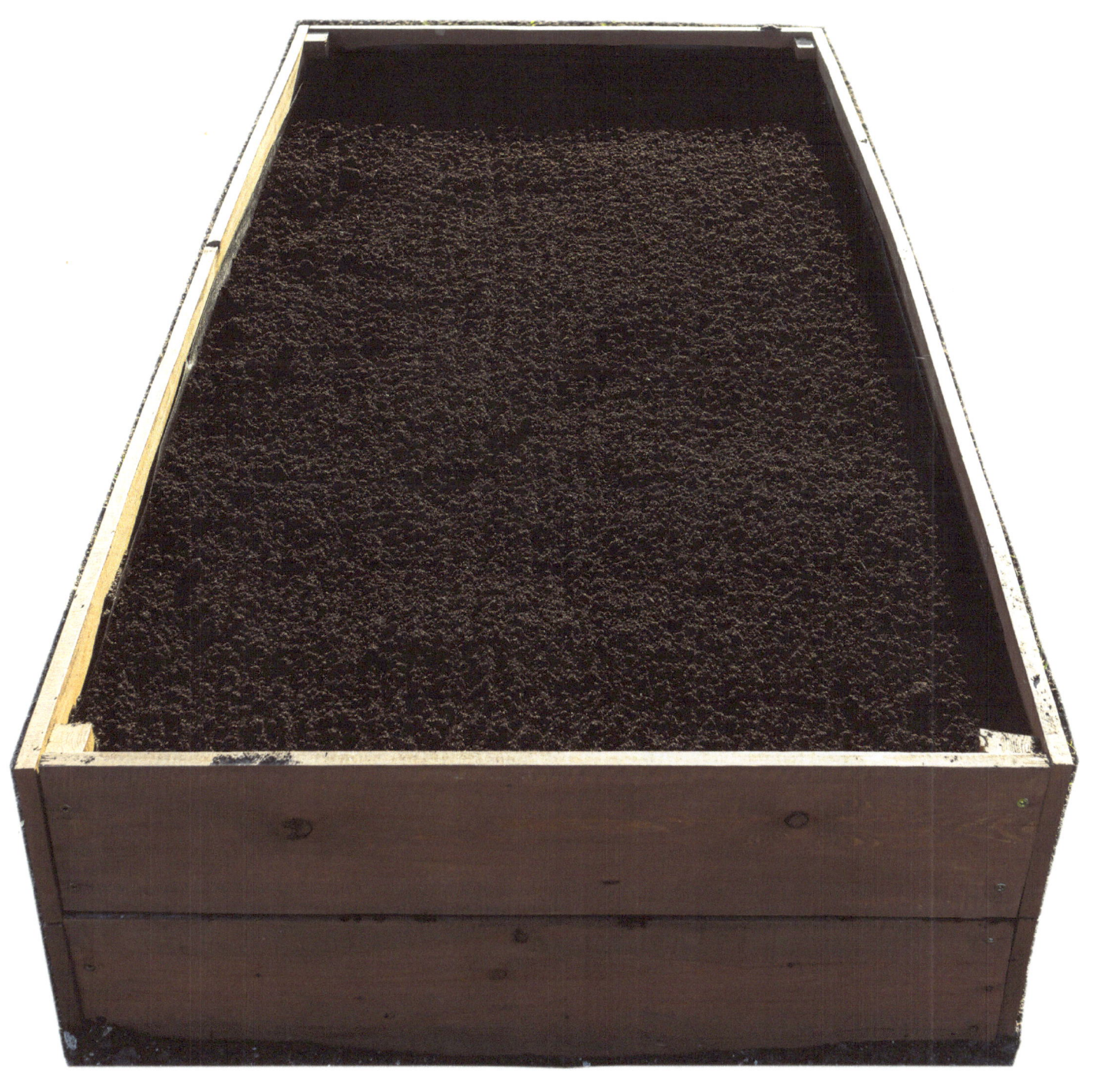

Special Thank You

Author's Acknowledgements

A special thank you to each of you for your ideas, inspiration, love, and support, to my colleagues: Vivian Vergara, Holistic Wellness Specialist, Sarasota, Florida, and Eleanor Tison, Co-Director, Green Mountain Center for Sustainability, Prescott College, Arizona; Kristin Little, close friend; and to my family: Shelley Ehrlich, Leah Wing, Deepika Marya, Jesse Wing, Monica Harris, Olivia Wing, and Elle Wing.

With Great Appreciation to These Illustrators and Photographers at ©Dreamstime.com

1evgeniya1
7active Studio
7vect0r
Abel Tumik
Adamnizol
Adisak Rungjaruchai
Adogslifephoto
Agami Photo Agency
Ahmad Safarudin
Ajafoto
Akinshin
Aleksandr Andrushkiv
Alessandra Rc
Alexander Babich
Alexander Konoplyov
Alexander Pokusay
Alexander Raths
Alexey Stiop
Alexoakenman
Alexokov
Allegro7
Allexxandar
Altitudevs
Altitudevs
Amnat Buakeaw
Anastasia Darii
Anastasiia Zabolotna
Anatoly Repin
Andegraund548
Andjelka Simic
Andreistanescu
Andreuma3
Andreus
Andrey
Andrey Golubtsov
Andrii Bezvershenko
Anemad
Anggraeni Sri Rahayu
Anico G. Enderle
Anikasalsera
Ann Moore
Anna
Anna Bergbauer
Anna Komisarenko
Anna Kucherova
Anna Lopatina
Anna Puhan
Anna Rusan
Anna Sedneva
AnnaMartinskaya
Annzabella
Araya Pacharabandit
Ariadna De Raadt
Arkela
Arloofs
Artem Efimov
Artex67
Artness
ArtoPhotoDesignoStudio
Artur Balitskii
Artur Kutskyi
Asetrovaann
Athapet Piruksa
Aviag7
Ayutaka
Azot Susila
Beata Jana Filarova
Beautifulblossom
Beinluck
Belusuab
Bert Folsom
Bianca Wisseloo
Biancaoddi
Blackphoenix1980
Bobyramone
Bohdan Skrypnyk
Boonmee
Bruce Macqueen
Canan Baris
Candace Schoner
Captivatinglightphotos
Casejustin
Castecodesign
Catarii
Charmaine Paulson
Chase Dekker
Chernetskaya
Chinook203
Chon Kit Leong
Chumporn Chophwan
Cleverson Felix
Cobia
Colin Buckland
Colorcocktail
Compsachen
Conceptcafe
Cookamoto
Corey A Ford
Corina Tintila
Cornelius20
Daisuke Kurashima
Daria Likhodedova
Dave Massey
David Cornelius
davidhoffmannphotography
Dayzeren
Debrahughes
Denis Kostroma
Dennis Jacobsen
Designua
Diana Eller
Diidik
Dipak Talati
Dj0038
Djvstock
Dmitry Krikun
Dmstudio
dorsetgirl2001
Dpimborough
Dracozlat
Duc Hong
dvoriankin
Eak Kem
Ekaterina Efanova
Ekaterina Glazkova
Ekaterina Mikheeva
Ekaterina Romenskaia
Elena
Elena Borisova
Elena Elisseeva
Elena Medvedeva
Eleonora Ivanova
Elina Yakhontova
Elizaveta Poroshina
Elokuu
Ennjee
Erik Zunec
Erika Norris
Erinphoto10
Ernest Akayeu
Ethan Daniels
Evamask
Evgeniia Parkhomenko
Evgeniya Grishkina
Ezumeimages
Famveldman
Farinoza
Fascinadora
Flashvector
Foster
Fotografiecor
Foxyliam
Francesco Pussumato
Frank Fichtmueller
Fredweiss
Freeprintbq
Friesart
Galina Malareva
Gary Gray
Georgii Dolgykh
Gijsvdabeele
Gl0ck33
Gloria Rosazza
Godruma
Golden Sikorka
Gorgulias
Grant Phillips
Grazia Natalotto
Green earth with leaves
Gribnick
Hanna Hryharenka
Harijanto Suwarno
Hartnett2007
Heather Jones
Henk Wallays
Honourableandbold
Hsiu Chuan Yu
Iamnee
Idey
Ievgen Melamud
Igor Tokalenko
Igor Zakharevich
Ihor Svetiukha
Ilja Enger Tsizikov
Ilya Golubev
Ilyakalinin
Imaginiac
Info11778
Inkdropcreative1
Inna Feshchyn
Inspirationupload
Ipolstock
Iquacu
Ira529
Iricat
Irina Belokrylova
Irinafotina
Irinav
Iryna Lukashuk
Iryna Zaichenko
Ivandzyuba
Ivansabo
Izanbar
Izonda
J2
Jairo Souza
James Mahan
Jan Havlicek
Jason Hindman
Jason Ondreicka
Jean Landry
Jedimaster
jeff waibel
Jehsomwang
Jenifoto406
Jianghongyan
Jixin Yu
Jminka
Joachim Berschauer
Joannatkaczuk
John Anderson
John Sirlin
Jon Bilous
Jose Mathew
Juan Moyano
Julian Popov
Juliengrondin
Justlight
Jyothi
Kamenuka
Kannan Sundaram
Karen Foley
Karl Ander Adami
Karl Umbriaco
Katarinochka
Kateryna Kon
Katrinshine
Keechuan
Kinek00
Kingan
Kitti Kahotong
Konstantin
Konstantin Gerasimov
Konstantin Kostan
Kostiantyn Kravchenko
Kotina
Kristof Lauwers
Ksena Shu
Ksenyasavva
Kurylo54
Kutukupretkw2
Leekkk
Lehmanphotos
Lesia Pavlenko
Lesichkadesign
Lhall49
Lianainasaridze
Lightkeeper
Liliya Shlapak
Lim Seng Kui

Acknowledgements

With Great Appreciation to These Illustrators and Photographers at ©Dreamstime.com

Liskonogaleksey
Llopartic
Lnsdes
Loflo69
Loreena
Lorna Jane
Luayana
Luis Echeverri Urrea
Lukaves
Lyubov Tolstova
Maart
Macrovector Art
Madartists
Maksim Bazarov
Maksim Pauliukevich
Mappingz01
Marazem
Margarita Vais
Margaritashi
Margo555
Maria Bobrova
Maria Kalashnik
Mariia Bogdanova
Mariia Domnikova
Mariia Sultanova
Marilyn Gould
Marina Vorontsova
Marinodenisenko
Mariusz Prusaczyk
Mark Hryciw
Martin Procházka
Mary Salen
Maryna Hlushko
Maryna Lahereva
Massimo Parisi
Mast3r
Max Lashcheuski
Md Khurshid Alam
Michael Gray
Michael Woodruff
Mike Monahan
mikrobiuz
Mila130189
Miloart
Mirecca
Miriam Doerr
Mogilevchik
Mohammad Shirani
Molekuul
Monika Adamczyk
Moonkin
Mr E J Wilde
Mr.siwabud Veerapaisarn
Mrjpeg
Mudwalker
Muradin
Nadezhda Shoshina
Nadiaforkosh
Nadiia Havryliuk Kharzhevska
Nahhan
Natalia Kazakova
Natalie Shmeleva
Nataliia Darmoroz
Nataliia Demydenko
Nataliia Vladymyrova

Natasha55
NatashaBreen
Natis76
Ncl
Nedim Bajramovic
Nehru
Nenilkime
Nerss
Nevinates
Nextmars
Nina Firsova
Nitipat Sadtasirichai
Nitr
Norbert Buchholz
Nurma Agung
Oksana Ermak
Oksana Smyshliaeva
Oksanabratanova
Oleksandra Martiukova
Oleksiy Kovalenko
Olena Danileiko
Olena Troshchak
Olesh
Olesya Turchuk
Olga Hmelevskaya
Olga Kriger
Ondrej
onnada srilawong
Orxpikdesign
Pairoj Sroyngern
Pascal Halder
Passiveaggressive
Patarajan
Pattarawit Chompipat
Pavel Naumov
Pavlo Syvak
Penchan Pumila
Peter Leahy
Phanuchat Prasertpol
Pheby
Philipp Schlüter
Photogallet
Picture Partners
Pimonpim Tangosol
Pisicasfioasa
Pisotckii
Piyapong Thongdumhyu
Pkzphotos
Pleshko74
Pnwnature
Polelya
Portraitquo
Potatushkina
Potysiev
Ppy2010ha
Pram Samnak
Premyuda Yospim
Pressmaster
Ptasha
Rainer
Raman Maisei
Ramilf
Rawpixelimages
Richard Carey
Rima Al Turk

Rinus Baak
Riverlim
Rob Jorg
Roberto Scandola
Robin Nelson
Rolandtopor
Roman Ivaschenko
Romana Anji
Ruslan Batiuk
Russieseo
Rvlsoft
Sabelskaya
Sarawut Samansup
Sarsmis
Sasha Kircanski
Sasha Kondr
Satheesh Rajh Rajagopalan
Sayda Nargish Parvin
Sburel
Scott Karcich
Seadam
Seamartini
Sean Steininger
Selentaoriart
Selvam Raghupathy
Sergey Kolesnikov
Serjio74
Setory
Siarhei Nosyreu
Siberica27
Sikth
Silvionka
Slowmotiongli
Snitovets
Soleilc
Somesun
Sonulkaster
Spelagranda
Stefano Ember
Stephan Pietzko
Stephen Moehle
Steve Byland
Steven Melanson
Stockeeco
Stu Porter
Styranets Oksana
Sumikophoto
Suriya Siritam
Sutichak
Svetlana Gardus
Svitlana Tereshchenko
Svitlana Vilhauk
Swee Ming Young
Takan Kaewswangsap
Tamara Didenko
Tanaphong Sattayamit
Tanyapeliustka
Tartilastock
Taseret
Tatiana Belova
Tatiana Pankova
Teekaygee
Teirin
Terrence Allison
Tetiana Gutnyk

Tetiana Kovalenko
Thanarat Boonmee
Themorningglory
Theresa
Thitinai Permsawat
Thongchai Anothai
THPStock
Tuja
Tural Mammadzada
Tyler Olson
Ueapun
Usersam2007
Vaivirga
Valentin Balan
Valentyn640
Valiva
Varvara Sharovatova
Vasyl Duda
Vasyl Kosolovskyy
VectorMine
Veronika Kornienko
Vgrebelskiy
Viacheslav Besputin
Viacheslav Dubrovin
Viennetta
Viktoria Kabanova
Viniciussouza06
Vismax
Vita30
Vitor Hugo Artigiani Filho
VittoriaChe
Vivilweb
Vladimir Ceresnak
Voislav Kolevski
Volha Paulava
Volodymyr Byrdyak
Volodymyr Markin
Volodymyr Ovcharov
Volodymyr Shevchuk
Wanlop Phuengyoi
Webpainterstd
Welcomia
Woodhouse84
Xsviatx
Yamasanphoto0708
Yamix
Yaroslav Borysovych
Yasonya
Yehor
Yelena Panyukova
Yin21205
Ylivdesign
Yodke67
Yodsawaj Suriyasirisin
Yolfran
Ys7485
Yuliia Inshyna
Yuliya Shevchenko
Yunaco
Yuri Arcurs
Yuriy Brykaylo
Zeechinchun
Zeninaasya
Zkruger

NutritioninaNutshell.com
Visit our website to find:

🌿

Natural Foods from the Tapestry of Life (ISBN: 979-8-9985183-0-0), referred to as the '*Tapestry* Resource Book' in this **ACTIVITY BOOK**

Nutrition Charts and Natural Foods Sticker Package

These educational materials are designed for educators and anyone studying nature and holistic health

🌿

Organic, regenerative farm store links available for traditionally-prepared, artisan-made natural foods

Copyright © 2025. All Rights Reserved.

www.ingramcontent.com/pod-product-compliance
Lightning Source LLC
Chambersburg PA
CBHW061155030426
42337CB00002B/17